12/13

Tinnitus Alleviation Therapy DISCARD

A Self-Help Program for Gentle and Lasting Recovery

Maria Holl, L.S.W., C.B.T.

Basic Health

The information contained in this book is based upon the research and personal and professional experiences of the author. It is not intended as a substitute for consulting with your physician or other healthcare provider. Any attempt to diagnose and treat an illness should be done under the direction of a healthcare professional.

The publisher does not advocate the use of any particular healthcare protocol but believes the information in this book should be available to the public. The publisher and author are not responsible for any adverse effects or consequences resulting from the use of the suggestions, preparations, or procedures discussed in this book. Should the reader have any questions concerning the appropriateness of any procedures or preparation mentioned, the author and the publisher strongly suggest consulting a professional healthcare advisor.

Basic Health Publications, Inc.
28812 Top of the World Drive
Laguna Beach, CA 92651
949-715-7327 ◆ www.basichealthpub.com

Library of Congress Cataloging-in-Publication Data

Holl, Maria
    [Tinnitus lindern. English]
    Tinnitus alleviation therapy : a self-help program for gentle and lasting recovery /
Maria Holl, L.S.W., C.B.T.
        pages cm
    Includes bibliographical references and index.
    ISBN 978-1-59120-364-3
1. Tinnitus—Treatment. 2. Self-care, Health. I. Title.
    RF293.8.H6513   2013
    617.8—dc23
                                        2013029911

Editor: Cheryl Hirsch
Typesetting/Book design: Gary A. Rosenberg
Cover design: Mike Stromberg

Printed in the United States of America

10   9   8   7   6   5   4   3   2   1

Contents

To all those who suffer from tinnitus:

*May this book provide the support
you need to help yourself.*

Foreword to
the German Edition

Tinnitus for the ear, nose, and throat specialist is a very dissatisfying and almost irritating syndrome, which he or she encounters on a daily basis. Difficult to diagnose and hard to treat, it requires a lot of patience and trust from both doctor and patient.

Being trained at a conventional university and influenced by orthodox medicine, it took me a long time and many years of intense work with tinnitus patients to learn not to search for one effective therapy or even *the* tinnitus therapy.

The fact that there is a wide range of tinnitus therapies available shows that there is no such thing as a unique and exclusive therapy. Treatment with ginkgo biloba extract, vasoactive agents, anti-inflammatory drugs like cortisone, infusions of lidocaine or caroverine, blockage of particular neural nodes, neural therapy, local anesthetics, acupuncture, sound therapy, laser therapy, oxygen multi-step therapy, or hyperbaric oxygen therapy—all these are therapies that can be perfectly effective in individual cases and help the patient to ease his or her tinnitus. However, none of them can claim to achieve an overall guaranteed or credible therapeutic success.

Only the patient can learn to live in peace with the tinnitus, to come to terms with it, and ultimately to even get rid of it. It is the task of the doctor and therapist with the help of friends and family to get the patient moving in the right direction, to help the patient help her- or himself, and to dispel fears.

It was only after my doctor's office had been inundated by a huge number of tinnitus sufferers and no help was to be expected from established psychotherapists or psychosomatic doctors of the region that I met Ms. Holl and learned of a completely different method of confronting tinnitus. Initial doubts turned into increasing confidence and finally into the conviction with which I support and share this concept. It is simple to carry out and has been successfully put into practice by a lot of patients over the years. A certain amount of imagination and trust in exercises, which appear almost too easy, is required; their aim is to provoke you into doing something for yourself and to start changing your former mis-programmed philosophy of life.

I sincerely hope that in using Ms. Holl's methods many tinnitus sufferers will learn to make peace with their tinnitus and to regard it as a stress indicator. To this end Ms. Holl has skillfully developed a self-help program in this book.

Herbert Philipps, M.D.
Ear, Nose, and Throat Specialist

Foreword to
the American Edition

For the last twenty-five years a dialogue has been taking place among those in the medical field about the essential role and function of the doctor and the patient, and about the healing process in general. In a healing process, who does what? How does healing actually occur? Does the healer "do" something to person seeking to be healed? Does did the patient "do" something to him- or herself? Does the healer "act" on the sufferer directly or indirectly? Does the practitioner facilitate the healing or is the healed transformed? What are the therapeutic actions that enable healing to work?

Tinnitus is a distressing, disturbing, psychologically and emotionally painful condition. For some, it is an inescapable affliction that disrupts relationships and life in general. Historically, the cause, or causes, of tinnitus have been subjects for speculation, with no clear and certain causal explanation emerging. The suffering, however, is plain and clear, and it calls on the practitioner of the healing arts to do something to help. But, on the whole, techniques and programs for amelioration of this condition have not been very successful.

Into this painful and difficult situation comes this book based on the extensive and many years work of Maria Holl in responding to this condition. The method described here, called Tinnitus Alleviation Therapy, answers the questions posed above by offering practices that the sufferer can engage in to help him- or herself, within a guiding structure created by the healer. The practices offered here have been tested over many years now with a large population of people suffering with tinnitus and the program is successful for many when applied by the sufferers in the way the practitioner recommends. This is hopeful news for the many people who suffer with this condition and have been unable to ameliorate it.

Ms. Holl regards tinnitus as a symptom—meaning that tinnitus represents the presence of a condition or state. In her view, this state is organismic and is made up of a complex interaction of external and internal forces and processes. Each person's tinnitus therefore represents a unique convergence of forces and processes that produced this symptom. Yet despite the vast and various causes of a person's tinnitus, Ms. Holl and others have found this program to work for many in the reduction of the symptom. Her understanding of the mode of action of this program rests on information derived from neurology, human energy systems, bioenergetic analysis, and clinical practice. She has developed a sophisticated model based on the interaction of these dynamics, both in the production of the symptom—tinnitus—and in its amelioration.

This model serves as the infrastructure for the self-enacted Tinnitus Alleviation Therapy presented in this book. It includes her theory about how the practitioner of healing is to interact with the person seeking to be healed. That comes through in the tone with which she addresses the sufferer and in the attitude she proposes that the sufferer adopt in relation to her- or himself and the suffering that is experienced. This is an important part of the healing process.

Tinnitus Alleviation Therapy inclines to the end of the continuum of healing arts that puts the initiative in the hands of the sufferer with minimal input from the practitioner. If the program works to alleviate the intensity of the symptom, then it has done its job, and the sufferer will undoubtedly be very grateful. Whether doing so addresses some of the underlying dynamics that Maria Holl has considered in fashioning this program is less important here, although she has seen broader transformative effects of the program itself. It may be that the sufferer will have to do more to address those issues by making changes in his- or herself or in one's way of life. For some this more extensive, deeper worker can be blocked by the symptom, by the tinnitus, which may feel too pressing to permit the therapeutic work to take place. These sufferers may say, "But, doctor, I can't think straight about myself with this terrible ringing in my ears!" These people too can be helped by Ms. Holl's ministrations as conveyed by the program in this book. And when that ringing can be reduced and with it the suffering it brings, we can all be grateful—healer and healed alike.

—Scott Baum, Ph.D.
President, International Institute for Bioenergetic Analysis

Preface

In 1996, a psychotherapist friend of mine told me about an ear, nose, and throat (ENT) specialist in her town who was urgently seeking help for a large number of his patients.

Since my children were growing up fast I had more time for new activities, so I rang up the doctor and we arranged to meet. On my way there I wondered how my skills as a psychotherapist, bioenergetic therapist, and practitioner of Western and Eastern alternative medicine could be of help to such a large established practice. Before I had even spoken to the doctor, I came to the conclusion that it could only be in the form of courses for the patients.

In our discussion it became apparent that all the patients for whom he was seeking help were suffering from tinnitus (a ringing noise in the ears). He had up to eight new patients with tinnitus every day for whom he had no conclusive, helpful therapy. After he had described the symptoms of their condition and some of the personality traits, I promised I would return in two weeks with a concept for a course.

After negotiations with an educational center of a hospital, I was able to organize a course there with help from the doctor's receptionist. The program combined a unique blend of therapeutic tools: bioenergetic exercises (a body-oriented form of psychoanalysis), self-massage, and inner exercises that combine visualization and special breathing techniques. To my delight, the general psychological well-being of some of the patients improved after only a few sessions, with the effect that their tinnitus lost its painful significance. We always had at least one person in every course who lost the ringing in his or her ears, as well as one who simply didn't see the point of the exercises. There were generally twelve participants in a course.

Those who took part in two consecutive six-month courses were particularly successful. For an entire year, they continuously practiced their exercises under supervision, learning new ones every two to three weeks. They also practiced these exercises regularly at home. These courses were the beginning of what eventually developed into a new approach for treating tinnitus that I call Tinnitus Alleviation Therapy (TAT). Presently, this method is being taught in individual and group courses by myself and other TAT-trained therapists in Germany and the Netherlands. Beginning in 2014, training classes will become available in the United States. As this unique approach in the treatment of chronic tinnitus continues to receive individual and clinical validation, as well as exposure through the German and American editions of this book, my hope is that it will become widely available to more people who suffer from this chronic yet common condition.

I would especially like to thank ENT specialist Dr. Herbert Philipps, whose determination to help his patients enabled him to accept this completely new therapeutic method. His commitment to this process has allowed me, with help from his receptionist, Karin Kallas, to conduct the courses.

At this point I wish to thank my teacher, Hetty Draayer, for her knowledge, her empathy, and her patience. The inner journey and the inner exercises that she taught me have played a vital role in developing the underlying skills needed to write this book.

I also would like to thank three trainers of the International Institute of Bioenergetic Analysis who were key people in my career: Susan Downe, Dr. Scott Baum, and Dr. Ron Robbins had a great impact on my professional career.

Finally, I also wish to thank my husband, Walter Holl, for his support, his understanding, and his faith in my skills, as well as my publishers, Dr. Werner Jopp of Oesch Verlag Publishing in Switzerland and Norman Goldfind of Basic Health Publications in the United States, for their appreciation of my therapy approach and for making it possible to publish the trans-Atlantic editions of this book.

If you have decided to read this book and do the exercises, we encourage you to show how these simple exercises can be a help to many tinnitus sufferers.

Tell your friends who also suffer from tinnitus about the exercises and talk to your doctors, so that these simple, unusual exercises, which are essentially thousands of years old, can once again unfold their therapeutic potential in our culture.

And lastly, many thanks to all who helped to create this book in both visible and invisible ways.

Introduction

You can benefit from this book, if . . .

▶ You suffer from tinnitus and do not wish to try everything conventional medicine has to offer.

▶ You suffer from tinnitus and have tried all or some conventional therapies which have not helped you.

▶ You do not suffer from tinnitus but work professionally with tinnitus patients and would like to try a new self-help program and learn it yourself.

Tinnitus is experienced as constant or recurring ringing noise in one or both ears. It is estimated that one in five people, or 36 million Americans, have the condition. The condition is difficult to diagnose and hard to treat. Part of the problem is that tinnitus is thought to result from a range of very different physical, environmental, and emotional causes, everything from poor circulation, high blood pressure, and wax buildup to persistent loud noise and stress. Some people have found relief from neural node blockers, masking devices, medications, local anesthetics, acupuncture, sound therapy, laser therapy, hyperbaric oxygen therapy, psychotherapy, and other coping techniques. The wide range of tinnitus therapies available shows that there is no such thing as a unique and exclusive therapy. None has proven equally effective for all those who are affected.

Tinnitus Alleviation Therapy

Tinnitus Alleviation Therapy, or TAT, is a unique method for coping with and recovering from tinnitus. It consists of a series of deceptively simple body-mind exercises that when practiced for fifteen to thirty minutes a day are able to remove the aggravating effects of tinnitus in eight of every ten people. Results from a randomized, controlled clinical study published in 2012 found scientific evidence that the Tinnitus Alleviation Therapy had a beneficial effect on more than 85 percent of the participants who followed the instructions and did the exercises (Kreuzer, P.M., et al. "Mindfulness- and body-psychotherapy-based group treatment of chronic tinnitus." *BMC Complementary and Alternative Medicine* 2012, 12: 235). The exercises are devised to activate your self-healing powers, as well as a self-awareness of aspects in your life that are contributing to your tinnitus and need to change. As a result, you are likely to find that Tinnitus Alleviation Therapy is not only valuable for relieving tinnitus but also for experiencing a healthier, longer, and more satisfying life.

How the Exercises Work

To a large extent, these novel exercises for the treatment of tinnitus come from China and do not work with the organs, muscles, or blood vessels, but rather with the energy system of the human body. It is the system through which our life energy, or *chi*, flows.

The specific exercises are derived from three types of exercise. Even though the types of exercise use very different techniques, their combination is far from arbitrary. They include:

1. Bioenergetic exercises: This type of exercise uses physical movements to help release suppressed feelings that can block energy flow and cause physical ailments.

2. Self-massage: A type of shiatsu-like massage that consists of stretching and massaging certain parts of the body in order to stimulate pressure points and open energy pathways, called meridians, to improve circulation and functioning of the glands, which in return has a positive effect on the immune system.

3. Inner exercises and special breathing techniques: Based on Taoist healing medicine, these exercises not only harmonize the flow of the life energy within the body but, over time, also help develop a new sense and a new awareness of the self.

The exercises help the natural flow of energy to circulate through the right channels and to stabilize our strength, by opening us up toward the earth. It is my belief that people who suffer from tinnitus have accumulated too much energy in the head, neck, and chest area and not enough in the pelvis, legs, and feet. For this reason, we start by doing exercises for the feet and legs, as well as the pelvis.

The exercises shift the focus away from the ringing in the ears and change the intensity of the tinnitus. (Think of tinnitus as being like a toothache: distraction helps; paying attention increases it—exceptions are rare.) Opening up the body toward the earth relaxes both the body and mind, reduces fear, strengthens self-confidence, and enables a new sense of self. Fears brought on by the tinnitus are reduced as well as other fears, such as fear of failure, agoraphobia (fear of open or public spaces), claustrophobia (fear of closed or narrow spaces), and fears surrounding one's health. The feeling of being controlled by tinnitus and other people slowly but steadily lessens. I could go on with this list. And it all depends on exercising daily for only fifteen minutes.

The exercises were devised for the modern person who works fifty hours a week, has two children, takes care of a house with garden, walks the dog, and visits the sick grandmother once a week. She or he can do an essential part of the exercises while waiting at the cashier, running for the bus, waiting for a family member, or being stuck in a traffic jam. The exercises are devised in such a way that with few exceptions they can be done everywhere without any auxiliary devices.

It is important to keep the following in mind before you start the exercises:

▶ The physical exercises are easy to do for anybody who doesn't suffer from physical ailments. However, if you are under medical treatment, talk to your doctor or physical therapist before doing an exercise that might be contraindicated or that could worsen your condition; say, for example, a slipped disk or a neurological problem.

▶ Always start exercising slowly and never overexert yourself. Push your limits but don't continue when you are in pain. With time your body will get used to the exercises and they will become easier. Always have a chair close by, so that you can sit down if you feel dizzy.

▶ The exercises slowly release tension in your body, and it can happen that tears may well up or your nose may start to run. This is completely normal and nothing to worry about, just keep some tissues close by. Take it as a sign that the exercises are working and continue doing them.

Note: Some exercises in the program are too powerful for pre-adolescents and should not be used unless under the supervision of an experienced therapist of TAT.

How to Use This Book

First of all, read the book from beginning to end and let it sink in. You may find the exercises strange, funny, implausible, scary, overwhelming, boring, stupid, interesting, embarrassing, exciting, thrilling, hope-raising, and so on. Allow all of these feelings. Every reaction is valid.

If you feel like putting the book away immediately, just do it. There are many ways to cure a medical condition.

But, if you want to read on and work with the self-help program, commit to these important next steps:

Step 1

Before every exercise session say to yourself: "I pledge to do these strange-seeming, very ancient exercises to help ease my tinnitus." You will feel reluctant once in a while, that's okay. Saying this phrase helps you recall the commitment you have made and carry on.

Step 2

Dedicate your exercising to a person who is important to you. Why? Another unusual idea! You suffer from tinnitus. A major element responsible for your situation is that you do nothing or not enough for yourself, yet for others you are available at all times. Ninety-five percent of all tinnitus patients I have met were very caring people, who would do everything for their family, job, and home. They themselves always got the short end of the stick. Dedicate your exercises to a person and give him or her permission to check whether you have exercised. This step may feel uncomfortable because you admit to someone else that you don't look after yourself. After three to six months, you can skip this step.

Step 3

Exercise fifteen minutes every day. Fifteen minutes is a must if you want to experience lasting benefit from the exercises. It sounds simple but if you have ever tried committing to an exercise routine before then you know what I mean. The excuses are endless and everything else is more important. Be good to yourself and do the exercise for fifteen minutes a day. Just get started. If you enjoy doing them and/or they bring relief, you can also do them for longer. Never do your favorite exercise on its own; all exercises work only in combination with each other.

The book is divided into twelve chapters, or lessons. Read carefully through each exercise before attempting it. It takes forty to sixty minutes to work through one lesson.

After you have completed the whole lesson with all its exercises, take a notebook and write down everything you can remember. The facts that you remember are the ones that are beneficial for you. This will vary from person to person. The body learns by itself and each person remembers the parts that are important for him or her. In this way one develops the right cure. There is no "right exercise" but one finds out in this way what helps. Experience shows that it takes about two weeks for the body to internalize new things.

For the next two to three weeks, exercise from the notebook for fifteen to thirty minutes daily. Then work through the next lesson, and all subsequent lessons, in the same way.

Now to Start

Set up your exercise area so that everything you need for practicing will be close at hand. It helps when first beginning the program to make sure you are alone. The room should be pleasantly warm. Dress comfortably (no shoes required), but wear socks if your feet are apt to get chilly. Find a suitable chair without armrests. Place a glass of water and tissues next to you, and sit yourself down. Now say to yourself:

> "I pledge to do these strange-seeming, very ancient exercises to help ease my tinnitus."

Remember to repeat this sentence before every exercising session. Change the commitment so that it suits you. Time and again you will be exposed to "new and unusual" exercises.

I wish you all the best. Enjoy the program!

1
· · · ·

Lesson 1

Wear comfortable clothes and sit up straight on the chair. Make sure your buttocks are warm. Remove your shoes and place your feet flat on the floor. Mind that the floor is warm.

A glass of water and tissues should be nearby.

Hold your head straight and tilt your chin slightly toward your chest so that your neck is a little stretched. (See figure 1.) Open or close your eyes, depending on what feels better to you.

Gently shake out your arms and imagine cubes or other geometrical objects falling out of your hands and fingers. Shake each arm for one to two minutes.

How weird, kid's stuff . . .

Pay attention to your posture: Is your back straight? Is your neck slightly stretched?

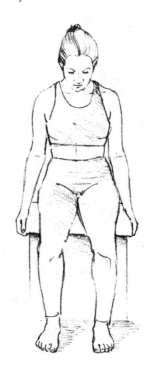

FIGURE 1.
Correct sitting posture.
· · · · · · · · · · · · ·

Shaking Out the Feet and Legs

Now shake out your feet and legs and let your chosen geometrical objects fall out of your feet. Shake each leg for one to two minutes.

Why cubes? Our autonomic nervous system doesn't understand words, only images. If I say, "let cubes drop out of your feet," the tension loosens. But if I say, "let the tension drop," nothing happens.

Check your posture once again: your back is straight, your shoulders are down, and your neck is slightly stretched.

Correct Breathing

Now place both hands on your lower stomach and breathe in. Do you notice how your stomach grows round and fat? When breathing out it sinks down and becomes thinner again. (See figure 2.) Breathe like this for two to five minutes.

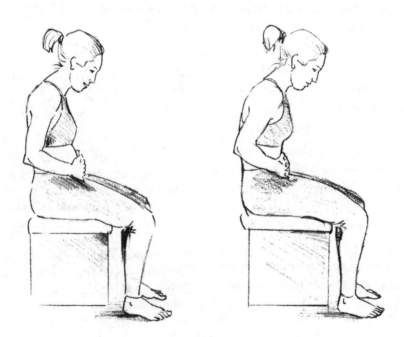

FIGURE 2. When breathing correctly, the stomach should expand on the in-breath (left) and contract on the out-breath (right).

With some people the stomach becomes thin when they breathe in and fat when they breathe out. That is the wrong way round. Practice breathing correctly in bed at night until it works automatically in everyday life. Practicing in bed will help you to go to sleep.

Now, feel your stomach with your hands while you practice. How does it feel? Is it hard or soft, warm or cold? If your mind starts to wander, observe the flow of your thoughts and then return your focus to your hands resting on your stomach.

If you are generally very tired, you will begin to feel your exhaustion now. Enjoy it and relax.

Now, place your right hand on your lower stomach. Hold your left hand like a bowl in front of your mouth, as if you want to spit.

Breathe into the stomach, which expands. Breathe out and imagine that your breath flows into your left hand. Slowly let your left hand sink down. Your breath in your hand flows down along your body.

This is an important exercise. You learn to control the direction of your breath. Your hands and feet probably feel warmer during this exercise.

Do this five times then take a short rest.

Now sit up straight and place your hands on your hips.

Feel if your hips are cold or warm. Take your time.

Rub, knead, and massage your hips until you can feel them and their warmth better. Take your time.

Occasionally shake out your hands, letting cubes or other geometrical objects fall out of them.

Massaging the Knees

Now place your hands on your knees. Observe how your knees and the hollows of your knees feel. Are they warm, cold, hard, soft, and so on?

You don't feel anything?

That too is normal.

They're not getting any warmer?

Sometimes you have to exercise for weeks before you feel anything.

Rub, knead, and massage your knees and the hollows of your knees until they feel warmer and are easier felt. Take your time.

Shake out your hands occasionally, letting cubes or other geometrical objects tumble out of your hands. Take a break and drink something.

Sit up straight on the chair again. If you have become restless through all this concentrating, walk around the room and have a stretch.

Then, sit down on the chair, sit up straight, slightly tilt your head forward, and let your shoulders drop.

Phew, it's so complicated.
Yes, that's how it is at the beginning.

Breathing Out Using the Hand Bowl

Repeat the breathing exercise just introduced to you in the exercise on correct breathing.

Place your right hand on your lower stomach and cup your left like a bowl in front of your mouth, as if you want to spit. Breathe into the stomach, which expands. Breathe out and imagine that your breath flows into your left hand. Slowly let your left hand sink down. Your breath in your hand flows down along your body. Do this five times.

What's all this about?
The body energy—the *chi* energy—is directed downward by the breath flowing down.

By doing this exercise daily we loosen the tension in the upper part of the body, which among other things provokes the tinnitus. All the tension is drained off downward. Now take a short break.

Observe yourself and ask: "How do I feel? Am I warm? Are my eyes watering? Am I taking the time to feel into myself?"

Don't be surprised if your eyes start watering. As you relax, the tear ducts open and tears may well up.

Massaging the Feet

Lift your right foot onto your lap. Find a position in which you can massage your right foot. Hold it in both hands and feel whether it is warm, cold, damp, or dry.

Slowly massage your foot from the heel to the toes.

> *This is really tiring. I am so stiff.*
> Shake out your hands occasionally letting cubes or other geometrical objects tumble out of them—slowly and calmly.

> *I am really exhausted.*
> If you have a strenuous job, your exhaustion will disappear due to these relaxing exercises.

After five minutes of massaging your right foot, switch to your left foot.

Drink some water and shake out your arms and hands. Massage your left foot also for five minutes.

Feel into your body: How do your hands feel? How do your feet feel? How are you sitting?

Your back is straight, your shoulders are dropped, and your chin is slightly tilted toward your chest.

Take a short rest.

Place your right hand on your lower stomach and your left hand like a bowl in front of your mouth, and repeat the exercise Breathing Out Using the Hand Bowl as described on page 10.

If your mind starts to wander, observe the flow of your thoughts and return to being aware of your breathing.

Breathe in like this for two to five minutes and keep concentrating on your breath. You are doing very well.

Lengthening the Little Toes

When you have finished this breathing exercise, raise your right foot onto your lap and rub your little toe. Then pull at your toe and imagine it growing longer.

That's funny. That's what children do.

Take a short rest.

Repeat the same exercise with your left little toe. Shake out your hands in between in the familiar way.

End the exercise as you like. If you have become restless from too much concentration, move or dance around; if you feel tired, relax a bit. You have done very well.

Now write down the exercises you remember from Lesson 1 and practice them every day for the next two to three weeks for at least fifteen minutes.

I can't remember all these details.
If you are an older person or have a bad memory, copy key-words of the exercises from the book into your notebook.

If you like to do a little extra exercise, imagine several times during the day that your little toes are growing longer. First they grow by two inches, then four inches, and at the end they are sixteen inches longer.

This exercise relaxes the ears.

2
....

Lesson 2

I t's good that you have found the courage to read on and maybe even go on practicing.

After you read through Lesson 2, set up your exercise area so that everything you need for practicing and to help you will be close at hand.

Every now and then remember the sentence you learned in the introduction: "I pledge to do these strange-seeming, very ancient exercises to help ease my tinnitus." From now on each lesson will be more "unusual" than the one before. This only means that these exercises need "getting used to," because we are no longer used to activating our self-healing powers. In times of emergency or when all external knowledge fails (doctors, medicine, science), our inner knowledge is reactivated and is made available to those who want to listen.

Take off your shoes, put on warm socks, and stand with your legs apart.

Your feet should be about the length of a forearm apart. Your toes are pointing slightly inward. (Don't let your feet point outward. In pointing them inward, we keep our power; in pointing them outward, we lose power.) Your knees are slightly bent.

This is really exhausting.

This posture boosts the energy flow in the legs.

Sometimes the energy flow is so high that the legs and even the whole body can start to tremble. Don't worry. If you straighten your legs, the shaking will stop.

Stand with your knees slightly bent for a couple of minutes and breathe into your pelvis.

Breathe out into your hand forming a bowl. The hand with your breath slowly sinks down along your body.

If you can't do the exercises in Lesson 2 standing up, sit on a chair as described in Lesson 1.

Massaging the Feet by Pressing Them into the Floor

Hold on to the back of the chair with your left hand and put your weight onto your bent left leg. Raise your right foot up on tiptoe. Massage the balls of your toes on the floor, using varying pressure. Start with your big toe and finish with your little one.

> *Ouch, that really hurts.*
> Try massaging a little softer. The ligaments and muscles of the toes are often very stiff.
>
> *Why do we massage the toes to heal tinnitus? After all, it's my ears that give me trouble.*
> By doing this, you are massaging the reflex points of the neck. Maybe you have already heard that foot reflexology can also help ease tension in the neck. The neck itself will be treated in later lessons.

Shake out your right foot from time to time. Don't massage it for too long; doing so could bring on cramps in your foot.

After massaging your foot, carefully curl in all your toes.

Now, use the floor to massage the tops of your toes. Be careful and do it gently, because it's even easier to get cramps when focusing on the top of the toes.

If this massage hurts a lot, then this is a good exercise for you.

However, don't overdo it and always massage the tops and the bottoms of your toes. When stretching you always have to stretch in both directions, otherwise you will end up being crooked. Shake out your foot at the end of the massage.

If you often twist your ankle, you should not shake out your feet. Please see a physical therapist and ask to be shown some exercises to strengthen the foot muscles.

If your foot hardly moves independently of your leg when shaking it out, you should move it very gently in order to loosen up the muscles gradually. Experience has shown that severe tension benefits most from soft massage; to relieve light tension, you can massage as hard as you find comfortable.

Keep massaging your right foot. Always finish one side before massaging the other, in order to properly feel the effect of each individual massage and exercise.

Next, tilt your right foot over onto its outer edge and. Using your body weight, massage it from front to back. Then shake out both feet. When shaking out your feet, please imagine that cubes, balls, or pyramids are falling out of them.

More nonsense . . .
Images are immensely helpful to relax the body. It will help you a lot in life if you keep this in mind. For example, you can use the image of the warm South Seas flowing through your shoulders in order to ease shoulder pains. Invent your own images. In the long run, you will be surprised how much they help you.

Go on massaging your right foot by pressing the heel into the floor. If you can still stand up, make sure to keep on bending your left knee otherwise the energy flow will be blocked in the knee.

That's far too exhausting for me.
It is very exhausting but it loosens the muscles in the leg. It's good to find out how far you can push yourself when exercising, but guard against being overly ambitious.

15

Finally, massage the inside of your right foot. Tilt your foot over onto its inner edge and press it bit by bit into the floor, starting from the heel and finishing at the toes. Your masseur or masseuse, so to speak, is the floor and the pressure you use decides on his or her force.

Finish this exercise by shaking out your feet and legs. Let the one shape of the three—cubes, balls, or pyramids, whichever best suits your imagination—fall out of each foot. Try shaking as long as it takes to surround yourself with a mountain of the shapes you have chosen.

Restoring Your Emotions: Part 1

Now sit down. Please take the time to witness how your feet and legs feel: Do they feel light or heavy, warm or cold, light or dark?

What's that good for?
Some people see a difference of brightness and light in the body. Try it yourself.

I don't see anything. I don't feel anything.
It's perfectly fine not to feel or see anything. If—like me in the past—you belong to the consistent non-feelers, it is important to "feel into the non-feeling."

As a help, I suggest you write a note with the sentence: "I allow myself to feel again, regardless whether it is painful, pleasurable, sad, shocking, or some other strong emotion."

Practice our special breathing technique. Inhale into your pelvis and exhale into the bowl formed by your hand, which then slowly sinks down along your body. Do this as described in Lesson 1 (page 8).

This little breathing exercise is one of the most important routines of the program. The breathing exercise and the self-massage help the breath once more flow through the entire body to keep it healthy, in the same way it does with babies.

Loosening Up the Ankles

Stay with the right leg. Begin by slowly moving your foot up and down, then to the right and to the left. Afterward, gently shake out your ankle with cubes or other shapes falling out of your foot.

Move your foot at least three times, up and down, then right and left, in between shaking out your ankle. The flexibility of the ankle is important not only for the backflow of the blood to the heart, but also for our flexibility in our own personal life and for the stability of our legs. The ankles are, in a manner of speaking, responsible for our stability in life.

Finish with shaking out your ankle and again feel the difference. To some, the difference will be extremely noticeable but others won't even know what there is to feel. For people who belong to the "non-feelers," it is unfortunately much more difficult to realize the results of the exercises. Often, they will notice the results in a changed behavior pattern, which obviously shows up much later than, say, a warm right ankle, immediately apparent after the exercise. If you are a "non-feeler," always use a hand to scan the appropriate part of the body for warmth and coldness.

You can also hold your hands or your legs parallel in front of you and check whether one arm or leg is longer than the other.

Releasing tension makes us taller.

Now scan your right foot with your hand: Is it warmer or colder? Does it sweat more or less or is it the same? How's the skin color: Is one foot rosier than the other? Find out the differences yourself.

> *This feeling and watching is really tedious, it keeps me from exercising.*
> It is important that you learn to feel yourself better again; therefore, you need to feel and watch your body consciously. It's one of the few opportunities to monitor your performance. The results will give you the energy to exercise daily for fifteen to thirty minutes. You need these exercises so that your tinnitus won't stress you anymore, or may even leave you.

Practice with your left foot now, in the same way you have done with the right one. After the relaxation break, write the exercises down in a notebook in order to better remember them. The more varied things you do with the exercises, the sooner they will become integrated in your life. By "varied things," I mean: read the exercises, write them down, make a drawing, do them, tell them to a friend, show them to others, laugh about them, and so forth.

As a treat you will now learn a simple but very effective exercise.

Leg Exercise for the Circulation

Sit on the chair, put your hands on your hip bones, and with the palms of your hands brush twelve times along the outside of your legs down to the little toes. At the little toes, continue to run your hands a little further into the air; this is called brushing out.

Feel into your hands brushing down your legs. Notice the structure of your legs, your trousers. The more your thoughts are with the exercise, in the feeling of your hands and in the respective body parts, the more effective this exercise becomes.

Brushing the outside of the legs stimulates the circulation. It's a good exercise for people who are grumpy in the morning, and it is particularly helpful for circulation problems.

The second part of the exercise is brushing up your legs, starting from your big toes to your ankles and along the inside of your legs up to your pubic bone. Do this also twelve times. Afterward shake out your hands.

This exercise helps the blood flow back to the heart and is good for people with vein problems. It relieves the veins.

Take a rest now. Drink a little water and breathe into the pelvis and out, using the hand bowl down along the body. Enjoy how your body feels.

Enjoy it? Now my legs ache.
If your muscles are very tense, it is possible that they now ache a bit. Sometimes you will have sore muscles after the exercises because the body power is activated. It means that the exer-

cises work and help you. Imagine your breath flowing into the areas that hurt. The pain will be more present but it will also leave sooner.

Most of your exercises will run as follows: you start with moving around in the form of walking, gymnastics, dance, or a self-chosen activity like gardening, cleaning windows, and so on. This helps to release stress, tension, and pent-up surplus energies, and gets them flowing.

The second part of the exercises is the self-massage where you learn to massage your body with your hands or with the pressure of the wall or floor.

The third part is the feeling or visualization exercises. They form the main part of the book and are the unusual elements here. At first these exercises will be novel for many of you. We all react differently to new things. Some of us are excited and think, "Great, something new, something different." Others react with anxiety, fear, or denial. Some feel embarrassed. If you belong to those who love a challenge, this book is for you. If you are more reserved toward new things, saying the following sentence might help you: "For my health I am willing to do strange and unusual exercises for fifteen minutes a day." Play around with the sentence so that it feels right for you. Giving yourself permission to do this could enrich your life.

Lengthening All Ten Toes

Sit straight on the chair. Your feet are shoulder-width apart, your neck is straight, and your chin is slightly pulled in to your chest so that the neck is a little stretched. Rub your feet against the floor so that they become the focal point of your awareness. Breathe into your pelvis and out into the hand bowl sinking slowly down along your body. Look at your toes and imagine them growing.

What's that supposed to mean?
The image of prolonged toes eases the tension in the foot and

the corresponding side of the body. During the next two to three weeks, your toes should grow longer and longer in your imagination. Start with a prolongation of two inches and step-by-step they grow until they are sixteen inches long. The body is surrounded by a layer of energy that reaches as far as sixteen inches from the skin.

Start with growing your right little toe. When you have accomplished this, you move on to the next toe to the left and imagine that one growing. You continue until you have reached your left little toe.

If you have trouble imagining this, put a sheet of paper under your feet and draw a sixteen-inch line to the left and right of each toe; they should not meet at the end. Draw two parallel lines per toe. In my courses, I compare these to clown's feet. The toes are as long as clown's shoes and you would fall over them if you had toes that long.

Now please change the breathing exercise in such a way that when exhaling the breath first flows into the hand, then along the body until it has passed the extended toes.

How can I exhale that long?
At the beginning you won't be able to do this. The first exhalation sinks as far as the pelvis, the second down to the knee, the third reaches the foot, and the fourth one passes the prolonged toes and flows away.

Keep exercising. You will eventually succeed in exhaling in one breath out along the extended toes. It's a steady progress. You don't need to force yourself. Have patience. I wish you joy and courage while exercising.

Participants of my courses are usually successful after exercising for three weeks to six months.

3
· · · · ·

Lesson 3

You have now reached Lesson 3. After you have worked through this chapter and have compiled your own program for the time to come, you will have learned a range of new exercises. If you notice that the diversity of exercises irritates you, put the book aside for a while and do only the exercises in Lessons 1, 2, and 3 until you get bored with them. You can also put a reminder four weeks ahead in your notebook that says something like "Continue working with the tinnitus book." After this chapter you will have learned enough exercises for some weeks.

If you are somebody who needs more "fodder," continue learning a new lesson every two weeks. You can allow up to four to six weeks between the lessons, but don't make the breaks any longer.

Remember to create a pleasant atmosphere for yourself. Make sure that the room is warm enough and that the phone won't disturb you. It's as if you are at home alone.

Observing Your Body

Start by standing up with your feet shoulder-width apart and your knees slightly bent. Close your eyes. If this feels unpleasant, stand looking at a corner you like in the room.

Now, your eyes look closely inward. Ask yourself: "How does the back of my head feel? Do I actually feel it? Is it warm or cold, or small or big? How does my scalp feel? How do my forehead, eyes, cheeks, nose, and mouth feel?"

I don't feel anything.
Firmly rub your face and hair several times with your hands. If you detect tension somewhere, rub this part a little more.

Now, direct your attention toward your throat, neck, shoulders, shoulder blades, arms, and hands. Do these areas feel warm, cold, dark, light, tight, loose? If you don't feel anything, rub your throat and neck, and tap your shoulders and arms as far as you can reach.

How should I tap?
Alternating the hands, gently tap the inside of your arm from your fingertips up to your armpit, over your shoulder, and down again along the outside of your arm back to your fingertips.

Next, direct your attention to your rib cage, chest, armpits, sides of your body, waist, back, stomach, and pelvis. Standing upright, inhale into your pelvis and exhale into the hand bowl, as described in Lesson 1 (page 10).
Repeat this three to ten times. How often you breathe depends on your patience.
If you don't feel anything, tap all these body parts, starting from the bottom up and back down again. Those of you who do feel something are of course also welcome to tap if you like.

How nice, slowly I am waking up.
Tapping awakens us.

Go on feeling and scanning your insides, pelvis, legs, and feet. Are your feet warm or cold? If you can't tell, use your hands. Scan these body parts before you tap them too.

My feet are cold.
If you have cold feet, use your hands to feel the point on your feet where the cold and warm areas meet. Massage this border between warmth and cold. The kneading can ease the tension there, which causes the cold sensation.

Restoring Your Emotions: Part 2

If you are someone who has trouble perceiving your body and this doesn't bother you, then skip the next couple of lines.

If you are a "non-feeler" and every now and then you get the impression that there is something missing in your life (such as love, pleasure, passion, sadness, joy), and you decide you want to feel again, then read through the next passage and add the exercise to your personal program.

Part of the "non-feeling" always shows in tension in the neck region or in a slightly tilted head. Ask somebody who sees you everyday: "How do I hold my head? Do I tilt it slightly to the right or to the left or do I hold it straight? Is my glance more turned up or more down?" With the information gained from this person, stand in front of a mirror.

Why do I have to ask somebody else? I can see all that by myself in the mirror.
We are in the habit of straightening up in front of a mirror. Our "normal" stance shows only when we feel unobserved.

While standing in front of the mirror, play around with the posture of your head. Lower it onto your chest, raise it up, tilt it to the right, then to the left. Do each movement three or four times; that's enough.

Nothing happens.
This is a tiny exercise to ease the tension in the neck. If you do it daily, you will feel more alive in the long run. If you are in

the habit of holding your head slightly tilted, only correct this while exercising. Otherwise, continue with your usual posture.

Now sit on the chair and take a rest. Resting always means to breathe using the special breathing technique into the pelvis and out using the hand bowl sinking down along your body (page 10).

Having done this five to ten times, write down the exercises you remember.

Always this tedious writing.
If it bothers you a lot, don't do it. But if, with a little persuasion, you could be made to do it, please write them down. You will memorize the exercises a lot easier, even if you never again check your notebook. And if you also do drawings, you will remember them even better.

Next, sit on the chair, place your feet shoulder-width apart, straighten your back, and tilt your chin slightly down. Move the ankle of your right foot to the right and to the left, and then up and down. "Nod" with your toes five to seven times. Subsequently, shake out your leg and foot, while imagining cubes or other shapes falling out of your foot. (See figure 3.) After shaking out your foot, place it flat on the floor. Breathe into your pelvis. Exhale into the slowly sinking hand bowl. Repeat three times.

Again this tedious breathing.
You will be asked again and again to watch your breathing in order to slow down your exercising. The flow of energy through your body will be strengthened doing this. When you concentrate on your breath flowing down your body, this energy will be shifted increasingly into your lower body regions.

I was always very irritated by these focused breaks, as if they kept me from doing the "actual" exercises. If you also react like this, make a face and say a couple of times: "This stupid exercise book, this silly. . . ." It helps a lot and eases the tension.

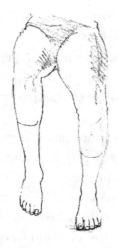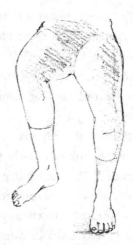

FIGURE 3. Moving the ankle in all directions (left) and shaking out the foot and leg (right) increases the flow of energy in the lower extremities.

Loosening Up the Knee Joints

While still seated, lift your right leg a bit and move it slightly out. You should be able to bend it without the chair being in its way. Bend your leg at the knee about ten to fifteen times and stretch it out again. Is your leg warmer now? Move it in slow motion, not as if warming up for gymnastics; do this movement very slowly.

> *Why so?*
> Moving slowly you feel intensely into your leg and knee, thereby filling both leg and knee with breath and energy.

Then, shake out your leg and imagine cubes or some shape falling out of it, at the same time following our special breathing technique (page 10). Now, you can take a rest from scanning and breathing.

Loosening Up the Hip Joints

Shift yourself a little to the right side of the chair so that half of your right butt cheek rests next to the chair. Lift the right leg and move it from the hip. The right hand rests on the hip joint. Starting very slowly and in slow motion, rotate the leg seven times to the back and seven times to the front. If your doctor or physical therapist contraindicated this or similar movements, please talk to one of them first!

Sometimes the hip creaks a lot or it seems not possible to do a round circle, but gradually the movement will become more fluid and rounded. The flexibility of the hip and the groin area is important not only for the physical motion, but also because all energy lines (meridians) run through this area and will be activated by the movement. Now shake out the leg and do the breathing exercise seven times. You can also use this time to rest.

> *These breaks make me really nervous.*
> Concentrate more on the breathing then the breaks will be work. Do you feel your right leg? And your left leg? Is there a difference? Is there no difference? Have a sip of water. Does it bring tears to your eyes or cause your nose to start running? This reaction often happens through tension release.

After a short rest, do the exercise with your left leg. Always do both sides before finishing the exercise.

The tension release sometimes lengthens the relaxed leg. You can check this while seated, by holding both legs parallel to the floor with the toes slightly tilted to the side so that the heels meet. Is one leg longer than the other?

When I do these exercises I notice a very definite imbalance between the already relaxed leg and the one still to be exercised. I feel virtually under compulsion to focus my attention on the other leg. Healing begins with attention.

You have now relaxed both legs. Walk around a bit and observe your walking; sometimes the loosening-up exercise changes the way you walk.

Resolving Dizziness and Tingling around the Mouth

Do you feel dizzy after exercising? It sometimes happens, partly because in doing the exercises we absorb more oxygen than usual. If you feel dizzy, stay seated, and kick and massage your right foot with your left foot. Then do the same to your left foot with your right one, and very often the dizziness will have already passed. Breathing more can also cause a tingling in your hands and fingers, and around your mouth. If that happens, put both hands over your mouth and nose like a hood, and for a little while breathe in your own air. There is too much oxygen in your body, and doing this small exercise brings in more nitrogen, which will stop the tingling. When you have done the exercises for a while, the tingling won't happen anymore because your body will have become used to the increased oxygen flow.

Sitting on the chair, put both hands on your pelvic bones and breathe into the pelvis. The pelvic area expands when you breathe in and becomes smaller when you breathe out. Imagine your exhalation flowing down without your "helping hand." Now grow your toes as described in Lesson 2 (page 19). Your exhalation sinks down along your body until it has passed the extended toes.

After this short rest of inhaling into your pelvis and exhaling along your body through your toes, once again sit up and position yourself comfortably on the chair.

Rock your pelvis slightly from side to side and feel the bones you sit on; they are called sitting bones. Starting from here, scan your revitalized legs, beginning with the right one. Feel into your leg and your right foot and grow your toes again, starting at the right little toe and finishing with the big toe. If you have practiced this exercise a few times, imagine your toes growing to be sixteen inches long.

What's up with these sixteen inches?
Our energy shell extends sixteen inches from our body. This invisible field is apparent in the polite distance we normally keep from each other. If someone comes closer than sixteen

inches to us, we perceive this as a lack of distance. Obviously, the acceptable distance between people may change in certain circumstances such as when riding on a bus or standing in a crowd.

After growing your toes, breathe again into your pelvis and out along your body. Let the breath flow out to the tip of the extended toes.

Growing Taproots Out of the Soles of Your Feet

Imagine that along the width of your right heel there is a sixteen-inch long orange taproot growing down. The root tapers off to the end and fine capillary roots sprout from it.

Don't strain yourself if this image doesn't come immediately. In order to stimulate your imagination, I suggest drawing a picture of it.

Two taproots also grow down from your big and little toes. The top of the taproot has a diameter of about two inches. Once you have successfully imagined these roots growing, there is one other taproot to focus on. This taproot is very important for tinnitus sufferers. It grows from the start of the kidney meridian, called the acupuncture point kidney 1, and is situated under your middle toe. Imagine growing a taproot from here, two inches in diameter and covered with lots of capillary roots. As this one is so important, you can grow it even two inches longer than the others.

Roots bring energy into your body and nourish you. At the same time they help you to release surplus energy into the earth. At times when you are very nervous, it can be helpful to imagine growing taproots, because the power and energy of the earth can flow back into your body through the orange roots.

You rearrange your energy body doing these unusual exercises. The composition of this body has an impact on your physical body. In eastern cultures even children know this; it is as obvious as the changing of the seasons. In our culture this knowledge is slowly returning. The pioneers of rediscovering old knowledge are always those people who haven't found help in the tried methods of our medical system. This makes it is easier for them to try something new and to devote the time necessary to learning something different from the traditional methods.

Now breathe into your pelvis and out through your legs, which you now imagine have turned into tubes; breathe further out through your feet and through the roots. Ask yourself permission to visualize this image. If it doesn't come to you, continue to breathe out along your body and along the roots. That is also fine.

Now do this exercise with your left leg. Then write it down in your notebook.

I thank you very much for your willingness to join me in being a pioneer for many other people. If you have the opportunity, tell other tinnitus sufferers about these exercises.

4

· · · ·

Lesson 4

You are now a quarter into the book. From now on, do the exercises of the program you have written down from the first three lessons for five to fifteen minutes before starting a new lesson.

We are now starting Lesson 4. If the chapters are too long for you, divide them into two to three units.

Sit on your comfortable chair. Your feet are comfortably warm (if not, put on socks). A tissue, a glass of water, and a towel are close to you. For this lesson you will also need a tennis ball or a massage ball.

How much did you exercise? Be honest with yourself.

Are you beginning to enjoy it? Do you feel the effects of the exercises in your daily life? Maybe you have become calmer or occasionally you say, "I don't want this," "No, I don't have time, I need to relax," or a similar sentence when people ask something of you. Gradually, you are becoming the focal point of your own life.

Reflect on what has changed in your life and write it down in your notebook.

Nothing has changed.
Do you doubt yourself? Do you have doubts about this book? Ask a person who lives or works with you what she or he thinks. Often we don't notice the changes in ourselves since we are always in our own company.

A woman in one of my courses had become a lot friendlier toward her clients but she only realized this when her colleagues told her: "You are now much nicer to other people."

It could be that at the moment the only benefit of the book is that you devote fifteen minutes of the day to yourself. At this point renew your decision: "I want to continue with the exercises!" Admit to yourself which days you didn't do your fifteen-minute exercise routine. Don't condemn yourself for it. Renew your commitment to exercise fifteen minutes a day. Once you have taken the hurdle of doing fifteen minutes daily, you will allow the exercises to take that space in your life, which is essential to improve your health in the long-term.

Maybe you are sick of my control: "How often have you exercised?" This control is part of the book. Many tinnitus sufferers have a problem with control. They want—no, they must—achieve everything and often 150 percent. And since that is impossible, the tinnitus sufferer usually chases his unattainable goal with a guilty conscience. You probably know the feeling. If not, start paying attention to how you react to control in your life.

More often than not control is experienced as particularly painful. I don't repeatedly ask those who are exercising regularly whether they are exercising; I ask the person who isn't exercising and who has a guilty conscience about it.

Expressing Rage

Sometimes the demands of life bring up rage and resentments. I suggest you buy a massage ball or a tennis ball and knead it firmly during or after such a situation. Then take a towel and wring it as hard as you can. Recall all the infuriating situations of the past. Scream out loud if you like while wringing the towel.

What will the neighbors think?
Show your anger; you won't harm anybody. But you will regain energy for life. Think of something to do to show your

anger and resentment, and remember that you won't harm anybody. Feelings of guilt and anger always belong together.

If you notice that you harbor many guilty feelings or a lot of resentment, add the anger exercise to your daily program. If the extent of your rage troubles you, talk with three people about it. It is important for you to hear that other people are also familiar with the topic of rage. Talk to a friend whose anger bothers you. Tell him or her about your own anger; you most definitely will be understood.

If at the end of the book or while reading it a second time, you are able to say, "I only exercised three times a week" without having a guilty feeling or "I exercised every day" without feeling especially elated about it, you have learned something very important. You have gained independence from the judgment of others.

Then begins a time when you are free to decide for yourself: Do I want to fulfill my duties 150 percent or is 100 percent enough or maybe only 80 percent is enough to feel good today?

After reading these lines you might increasingly be confronted by your feelings of guilt and your dependence on the judgment of others. Don't change your reactions when you notice your dependence.

Observe yourself amicably and neutrally and don't judge your behavior. Accept yourself as you are and be patient with yourself. A change in behavior starts from the inside, like the growing of a plant. Don't force anything, otherwise you will only be subject to a new restraint.

Today, start your exercises standing up. Stand next to the chair with your legs apart. Position your feet about fourteen inches apart. Your knees should be slightly bent. Move up and down a little to find the stance most comfortable to you. (See Figure 4 on the next page.)

Standing in this position with a slight bend in your knees is very important for soothing your tinnitus. Although this stance may be perceived as difficult, it actually loosens up the legs. In my courses, I suggest putting a note on the bathroom mirror to remind yourself to brush your teeth with knees bent. That way every day you can

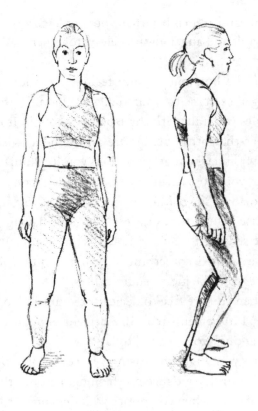

FIGURE 4.
Standing with the
knees slightly bent
is an easy way to
loosen up the legs.
Front view of body
(left), side view
(right).

loosen up the muscles in your legs and increase the energy flow in
your legs and feet without spending extra time on it.

Loosening Up the Pelvis

Standing with your legs apart, move your pelvis forward when
breathing out and back when breathing in, like a swinging ship in an
amusement park. Start very slowly.

If you are under medical treatment for physical problems, only
exercise as your doctor or physical therapist has advised you to. If
you aren't sure, show the exercise to the medical provider and ask
him or her whether you can do it.

I can't move my pelvis at all. It's stiff!

Put your right hand on the front of your pelvis and your left one on your back. Use the pressure of your hands to move your pelvis very carefully forward and backward.

First do the exercise without watching your breath. This exercise is particularly important for you if your pelvis, back, and hip joints seem tight.

An inflexible pelvis blocks the energy flow into the lower parts of the body.

Slowly your movements become faster and stronger. You feel as if you are trying to hit somebody with your pelvis.

Maybe you notice that your toes are getting very cold. Coldness is always a sign of fear. Maybe you think you aren't afraid. Even if you don't feel frightened, coldness often occurs when we do something new or unfamiliar for the first time. If your toes are cold, massage them until they become warmer, as shown in the Lesson 2, Lengthening All Ten Toes (page 19).

Activating the Warmth of the Body

If your toes don't warm up, rub, knead, and scratch your neck and the hairline. The "heating coils" of the body run through this area. If you still remain cold, rub, knead, and scratch the sides of your body from your armpits down to your hips. If you were in front of a mirror, you would look like an ape grooming itself.

If your hands get tired, shake them out, imagining cubes, balls, or triangles falling from your fingers. Choose the three-dimensional shape that suits you best.

If you often feel cold, this scratching and rubbing exercise is an excellent way to overcome it.

Whatever next?
Decide yourself which exercises you want to do and for how long. You may say, "I want to exercise for fifteen minutes" or "for 30 minutes."

Compile your own program. If after a while you become faster, add another exercise. If you take longer, take one exercise out. At the beginning, you need more time for the exercises but gradually you can do more in the same period of time. Don't rush yourself. To do one exercise with concentration is worth more than doing many without inner participation. If you notice that you can't stand up any longer, just sit down.

Massaging the Pelvis and Groin Area

Now start with your pelvis. Rub and massage your whole pelvis, front and back. Then take a rest. Inhale into your pelvis and exhale down along your body until your breath reaches below your feet. Do this several times.

Continue with the massage. Focus particularly on your groin area, which is situated between the pelvis and the thighs. The groin is the gateway to our legs. Massage the area using small circular movements.

It hurts.
Massage more softly.

I can feel big lumps.
If you are worried, see your doctor.

Massage first your right side, then the left. Our exercises frequently move from right to left. In the inner exercises of Taoist medicine, the energy of the day flows from right to left.

My hands are tired.
Shake out your hands as usual.

Already done.
Super!

Massaging the Hip Joints

Now we turn to the sides of the pelvis. Massage your hip joints.

Can't do it, there's only skin and bones.

Take a tennis ball or a massage ball and stand sideways against a wall. With the ball at the height of the hips, use your hips to press the ball against the wall or door.

Keep hold of the ball with your hand and slowly move your pelvis. You decide how hard to press. It sounds complicated but it isn't.

The exercise regenerates the whole body because all energy vessels (meridians) of the body pass through the hips.

When you have finished with the right side, sit down and feel the difference to the left side. It can be significant but doesn't have to be.

Stay seated, rest a bit, and shake out your arms and your hands (with three-dimensional figures), then take courage to start the left side.

I get all tired.
The hips carry a lot of tension and we always get tired when old tensions are released; it can feel as if we have just finished a mountain hike. Choose your time to exercise so that you have some time to sleep or rest afterward. If you find it hard to fall asleep, view the fatigue you feel after the exercise as a gift and use it to help you sleep.

Sit down when you have finished massaging both hips. Your pelvis now feels very alive.

Write down the exercise. Note what you remember and how it felt; for instance, did your pelvis feel warm or cold, dull or alive? Start "feeling." People with tinnitus frequently have reduced "feeling" but they "think" very fast. Start asking yourself from time to time: "What do I feel right now?"

Sit on the chair—legs about eight inches apart—and put your

hands on your pelvis. Breathe in, the pelvis expands and widens; breathe out and it narrows.

Some people do the opposite. If it is true for you, make this exercise the most important priority for the next two weeks. Breathing in makes the stomach expand; breathing out flattens it!

The breath is the foundation of our existence.

Now the unusual exercises start.

Wiping Out the Pelvis with a Cloth

Imagine cleaning the inside of your pelvis with a soft and cuddly white cloth, as if it were a big bowl. You wipe all sides, from the right to the left, from the back to the front, from under your groin to the iliac crest to the genitals, and so on. Wipe out your whole pelvis very lovingly and attentively. All the while your hands rest on your pelvis and perceive the whole area.

When you have finished wiping, breathe into the pelvis and out into the hand bowl that sinks slowly down along the body. Breathe seven times.

Cleaning the pelvis with a white cloth and breathing into the pelvis and out using the hand bowl along the body (page 10) are important exercises.

It seems very strange.
Yes, it's novel and it comes from another culture. To begin with, they are unusual exercises.

In your imagination use a pink cloth now and repeat the exercise with a pink cloth.

Whatever for?
Pink is good for the nervous system and calms it. If you are often nervous and afraid, use the pink cloth first when doing this exercise.

The Pink Breath

Now imagine your breath turns pink.

> *I hate pink.*
> Pink is a very important color in our life. If you dislike pink, buy some pink flowers from time to time to get used to the color.

Fill your whole pelvis with pink air and breathe out into the hand bowl with pink.

Do the breathing three to seven times. You can do these exercises also when lying in your bed. It is important that you breathe into your pelvis and out down along your body. If this proves difficult to do, start by doing it sitting down.

This ends our exercises for today.

5

Lesson 5

You might feel like changing the order of your personal exercise program once in a while. If so, do as you wish, but always start your exercises with one for the legs and feet.

Stomping

Exercise standing up. As usual, your feet are kept parallel and shoulder-width apart.

Stomp around and imagine you are in prehistoric times, trampling the warm, damp, dirt floor in your hut. Sink at least eight inches to the ground. If you have no neighbors below, stomp hard, so that the glasses in the cabinet start to clink. If somebody lives downstairs, stomp quietly but firmly with your whole foot.

It is important that the heel, middle foot, and toes touch the ground. Often we prefer touching the ground merely with our heels or toes.

Tread the "clay" slowly and firmly, paying a lot of attention so you don't slip.

Circle three to five times around the table and chairs. Stomp around the room. At the beginning you'll probably feel a little stupid. Feeling stupid helps the healing process; the more stupid the better!

Loosening Up the Legs

After stomping around, stand in front of the chair and shake out your legs and feet. Start slowly, first with your right leg, then with your left. If this feels uncomfortable, massage your legs and feet.

Afterward put both feet flat on the ground and alternate lifting the heels on each foot. Slowly pick up speed. After your muscles are warmed up, you can tremble very fast with your legs.

I can't tremble with my legs.
If you can't tremble with your legs, do the exercise three times for one minute. If possible see a massage therapist to get a leg and full-body massage. It can take time to release the tension of the leg muscles, particularly for men.

After loosening up your legs, start moving your upper body and spine like a contortionist—twist, wriggle, and bend your spine in all directions.

After you have moved like this for a few minutes, stand with your feet shoulder-width apart and your knees slightly bent.

Swing your pelvis gently back and forth. Do this five to ten times and finish with your pelvis tilted backward and your perineum pointing down.

You might need a mirror to check the right position, usually we tilt the pelvis slightly too much forward or backward. Check in front of a mirror whether you have tilted the pelvis too much. Bring it to the middle. You can also do this in everyday life whenever this exercise springs to your mind.

Breathe into your pelvis and out into the hand bowl slowly sinking down along your body (page 10).

Why this breathing technique?
We obtain the most energy when breathing deeply into the pelvis. The breath finds its optimal space because the lungs can expand and there is more volume for the inhalation. The breath directed downward fills you with energy and it helps

you to perceive situations better. If you succeed in learning to first look after yourself and only then use your leftover energy to help others, it will be a big step toward healing yourself.

My relatives will think I am selfish.
Don't worry. It's not that easy to become an egoist. It's more often the case that partners of tinnitus sufferers appreciate the patient paying more attention to him- or herself, as this reduces the inner scream (tinnitus).

Grow taproots out of the soles of your feet as described in Lesson 3 (page 28) and root your feet while standing upright. This exercise is an essential part of the program; therefore, it is important to practice the exercise daily until you feel comfortable with it. Don't give up if you don't succeed at the beginning. Keep on exercising and draw a picture of it every day. It's worth it.

Stand with rooted feet and slowly let your head sink to your chest and then lower still. Breathe into your pelvis and out through your feet. Your head can sink down until your fingers touch the ground. (See figure 5.)

If the ringing in your ears becomes louder, bend over slightly. The head hangs like a bell.

Since the tinnitus sufferer usually pays little attention to him- or herself, this is an excellent exercise to imagine you bowing down to yourself.

What's that supposed to mean?
People with hard shells often carry a lot of criticism and "covert" resentment for themselves, so that when they start to honor themselves they take a giant step toward healing.

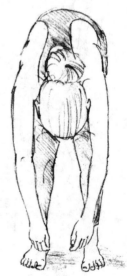

FIGURE 5. Bowing over until the fingers touch the ground helps loosen the spinal discs, as well as promotes appreciation for the self.

If it seems strange to bow down to yourself, do it without the image and concentrate on the physical side of the exercise.

After your head has slowly sunk down, completely straighten up again in slow motion—this is a very good exercise for the spinal discs.

When standing upright again, root your feet again on the four spots as described before in growing taproots from the soles of your feet. Breathe into your pelvis and out through your feet and the roots. When you have succeeded in directing all your energy toward the roots, slowly start stretching back.

Stretching the Body: Part 1

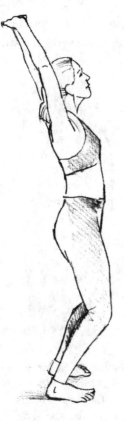

Lift your arms and pull up your hands so that you feel the tension in your stomach. Pull your hands back as far as they go. Breathe into your pelvis and out through the roots on your feet. (See Figure 6.)

How can I do that on top of everything else?
It only takes a little practice. At the beginning it might be difficult to do it all at the same time. Don't push yourself. Only stretch your arms and pull them back, and then gradually add the breathing.

Repeat this stretch a couple of times and see if your sense of well-being improves. If so, add the exercise to your program.

If you have the feeling it doesn't help you at all, just leave the exercise out. Opinions are divided on this exercise; some love it, others hate it.

FIGURE 6.
Stretching the arms.

44

Take a little rest. Sit down. Breathe into your pelvis and out into the hand bowl sinking down along your body. Now you can write down the exercises of this lesson.

Write down everything you think is important, even if it doesn't seem related to the exercise. You might pin a note with keywords on a prominent spot to remind you of an important thought. For example, something like "I am always ready to honor myself" might be helpful.

My suggestions mostly irritate at first. Maybe you think, "What nonsense," "What a stupid book," or "She's lost her mind." Allow these thoughts, write them down, say them out loud. If you "respect" anger, something new will happen and this is what counts. Sometimes change only happens through anger. You could even say that change happens only when we face our inner darkness: our unconscious.

Now that you are sitting down, spread your legs shoulder-width apart.

> *I can't do it.*
> People—both male and female—who have been sexually assaulted find spreading their legs to be a challenge, even an insurmountable obstacle. This may also be the case if your upbringing was very hostile to sexuality.
>
> If this is a problem for you, leave your legs together; it's not so important that you have to force it. Listen to your refusal. Doing so often tells you more about who you really are.

With your feet shoulder-width apart—or not—place your hands on your groin, the body's gateway to the legs.

Keep your hands on your groin for several minutes and breathe in and out using our special breathing technique (page 10).

Wiping Out the Pelvis and Groin with a Cloth

Slowly massage your groin—either all over, or first right and then left—nip, pinch, and rub your groin with your hands.

Using your index, middle, and ring finger massage your groin area in small circular movements, starting on the outside of your pelvis down to the middle of your pubic bone.

Disgusting. You don't touch yourself there.
Whenever you feel shame, please be kind to yourself; allow yourself to feel a little more ashamed each time. On the other side of shame lies freedom, so "feel ashamed."

Move three to four times back and forth from your groin to your pubic bone. Shake out your hands in between.

Take a little rest, root your feet, and grow taproots from them as described on page 28. As learned in Lesson 4, clean your pelvis with a soft white cloth (page 38).

Then, very carefully and lovingly, clean your groin and your pubic bone. In your imagination you take a soft white cloth and, beginning on the outside right of your groin area, wipe under the groin, then under your pubic bone and under the left side of the groin, until you reach the outside of the pelvis. Do this inner cleaning five to seven times. The exercise is important because the opening of the groin has a lot to do with our "standing in life." Our upper body is connected to the earth through our legs and feet, only if the groin area is open.

If you are sometimes scared, cleaning under the pubic bone is a good exercise, because this is where fear is at home.

Turning the Legs into Light Tubes

In your imagination take the cloth and reach into your right leg, which has turned into a wide tube of light.

My leg is not a light tube.
It doesn't matter. You open up your energy body with this image. The exercises don't describe the world of flesh and blood; they are effective in the reality of our energy body.

With the cloth, wipe the inside of your leg tube, up, down, and sideways, and slowly move down to your right foot. The foot feels brighter and more open.

Wipe the inner walls of your foot and toes—a lot of work. After you have cleaned your whole leg, let your toes grow as described in Lesson 2 (page 19).

When you have finished with the right side, breathe deeply and observe how your right leg feels.

Imagine an open tunnel running from the first digit of your right little toe to the first digit of the next toe, and so on up to the big toe—like creating an open arcade in the small bones much like the arcades found in southern European cities.

Turn to your left leg now. When you have finished with your left leg and foot, build a passage through the first digits of your toes from the little one to the big one. There's a beautiful light passage now running from left to right through the first digits of your toes. Feel into it.

I feel something, I feel nothing. Both are all right.
Enjoy a little rest.

Please exercise every day. Resolve to exercise for short periods; that way it is easier to get started.

6
· · · ·

Lesson 6

I would like to thank you for your courage in committing to doing such unusual exercises on a daily basis.

If you do not exercise daily, there's no need to be hard on yourself. It is difficult enough to exercise once in a while, to take time for yourself. Pay yourself a compliment for trying and resolve to do the exercises daily.

Working with a Display

Choose a symbol for your desired recovery. It could be beautiful flower, a stone, or the image of a loved one. This symbol will remind you daily to do your exercises. Put the symbol you have chosen in a spot you often look at. Whenever you see it, you will be reminded of yourself, your health, and your exercises. I make use of this to remind me of things that are important in my life but which I tend to forget. You can call this symbol a display. I consider it very helpful for personal training. You can use it as a reminder for all the important things in your life.

Read this lesson through once and observe your thoughts and feelings.

I don't get the point. Very strange, I'll skip that one.

Observing your thoughts and emotions is also part of the exercising program.

I don't have feelings.
Write down your thoughts and feelings in your notebook if you don't want to scribble in this book.

We don't have any problems with observing our positive thoughts and feelings. When we're happy, we feel recognized and good; we're more apt to think: "This book is good, it works like a charm."

Dealing with Negative Emotions

We get into trouble when we have to deal with negative thoughts and feelings. Maybe you think: "stupid book" or "these exercises are for babies." Maybe you feel ashamed because you think all this exercising is pointless.

You want to stop. You don't want to go on practicing. All of a sudden you come up against your anger; your helplessness; your difficulty in learning something new, thinking something new. You have reached your limit.

If you don't have these "negative" emotions, just skip this exercise and go to the next. If the negative emotions appear later, come back to this exercise.

Taking your frustration seriously by writing it down, by grumbling and nagging and complaining about this book, you start your recovery. You are frustrated about something you do for yourself, yet you don't stop yourself doing it. That's new. You keep on working for your boss feeling frustrated but for yourself often you don't.

Stretching the Body: Part 2

You are standing. As usual, your feet are kept parallel and shoulder-width apart. Your knees are slightly bent.

It feels uncomfortable.
This exercise puts the body in stress, which slowly and steadily relaxes the leg muscles.

Intertwine your fingers, raise them above your head and turn your palms to the ceiling. (See figure 7, left.) Stretch your hands up as if reaching for the ceiling. Do this three to four times.

Release your hands; slowly drop your arms and hands, and shake them out. Imagine three-dimensional shapes falling out of your fingers. In front of your inner eye, heaps of cubes, or something similar, start piling up under your right and left hands.

That's odd.
If you have problems with inner images, don't push yourself.

Raise the folded hands up above your head, and pull them to the far right; you should feel the pull along the left side of your body. (See figure 7, right.)

Breathe in and pull with your arms—the left side grows bigger. Breathe out and decrease the pull on the left side—the side shrinks again.

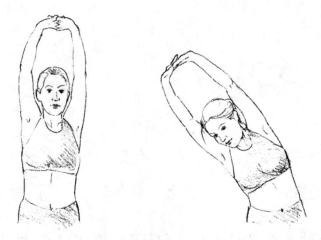

FIGURE 7. Stretching the sides of the body.

Don't do this more than five to ten times! You easily get sore muscles when stretching.

Let your arms and hands slowly sink down and shake them out. Scan both the right and left sides of your body.

I don't feel anything. I feel all asymmetrical. I'm all hot.
These are some of the reactions possible. All reactions are okay.

Raise the folded hands up and push your palms upward. Pull your arms and hands to the left. Breathing in, you pull; breathing out, you let go. Inhale and the right side curves out, exhale and it shrinks again. Stretch five to ten times.

If the ringing in your ears gets worse, do the exercise for growing toes from Lesson 2 (page 19) and breathe out using the hand bowl (page 10).

If your breath falls down all by itself, you can stop using the hand bowl. You can now do this exercise anywhere you are, whenever you want. The same is true for all the inner exercises.

You have finished stretching the sides. Fold your hands, pushing the palms out, and stretch your hands forward toward a wall or door. (See figure 8, left.)

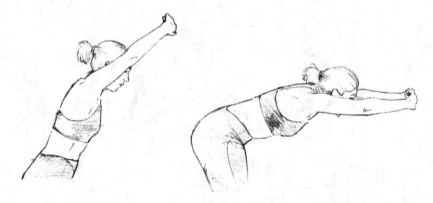

FIGURE 8. Stretching the backside of the body. Angle the arms up and push the palms outward (left), then bend and stretch the arms and hands.

Bend your body downward 90 degrees and stretch your hands to the front, keeping them at eye level. You can feel the stretch on the posterior side of your body. (See figure 8, right.)

Breathe in and out, three to five times, and slowly straighten up. Shake out your arms and your whole body.

> *That really hurts.*
> If you don't feel the stretch, this exercise is not important for you. If you tend to be stooped or you feel the cold easily, this exercise could be helpful.

The final stretch is to the back.

Fold your hands behind your back this time, palms pointing down, and stretch down toward the floor. (See figure 9, left.)

Then stretch your hands backward and upward as much as possible. When you do this, bones might creak or even adjust. (See figure 9, right.)

> *It's too tense; it's not possible.*

Do this stretch three to five times. Release your hands, move hands and arms, and shake out your whole body.

FIGURE 9. Stretching the back. Stretch hands backward and downward (left), then backward and upward (right).

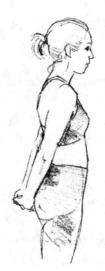
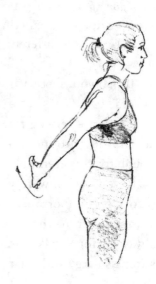

That was a really exhausting exercise.

Sit down and observe your body. Sit comfortably on the chair with your feet in warm socks (without shoes) and your back straight and upright.

Next to you are tissues and a glass of water. Drinking water is soothing, and you might need the tissues because your eyes may start to water after the exertion.

Breathe into your lower pelvis, grow your little toes, and let the breath fall down along your body. Breathe like this for some minutes and take a little rest.

Write the exercise down in your notebook, then feel into your pelvis.

> *I can't feel my pelvis.*
> Put your left hand on the front of your pelvis, and your right one on your back. Breathe into your pelvis and out along your body, through your legs and feet, and a further sixteen inches into the ground. It's as if you are completely permeable. Breathe like this a couple of times.

Scan whether your feet are cold or warm.

> *I don't feel anything.*
> You don't feel anything? Don't worry. Everybody's physical awareness is different, that's normal.

Touch your feet with your hands and feel whether they are warm or cold.

If you are very agitated, put on a CD (compact disk) and dance around, jog around the block a couple of times, or prepare the dough for this evening's pizza before proceeding with the exercises.

If you feel inwardly quiet, forget these suggestions and stay seated. It is important to move around when you feel restless. Don't sit down before the agitation has gone away. In times of stress I always go for a walk. Discover for yourself how best to get rid of your surplus energy and what is possible in your environment.

Growing Roots from the Sitting Bones and the Tailbone

Sit on the chair and place your hands on your pelvis. Breathe into your pelvis and breathe out along your body.

Put your weight onto your right side and sit on your right buttock. Feel the bone; this is the sitting bone.

Using small circular movements push the bone into the chair, forward and backward, until you become more and more aware of it. Now imagine an orange taproot with many small capillaries growing from it, through the chair and sixteen inches into the ground.

> *What's that supposed to mean, roots into the ground?*
> The body releases tension with this image. You feed the earth, so to speak, with your tension.

> *But I live on the tenth floor.*
> Don't worry. The tension will find its way into the ground.

The taproot should be at least three inches in diameter and should taper toward the end.

This exercise increases your inner stability and roots you in the ground. You will become more independent of other people's moods and opinions, and more stable in yourself.

Now shift your weight onto your left buttock and keep watching your breath. Are you still breathing into the pelvis? Is the exhalation still falling down to the ground?

> *What are you thinking? Nobody can do all that at the same time.*
> At the beginning it is nearly impossible to do two or three inner and outer exercises at the same time, but after a while you'll manage. To focus on two or three things simultaneously sharpens your powers of concentration. If you can concentrate only on one thing at a time, don't get flustered. Keep doing the one thing, and all at once you'll notice that it is easy to concentrate on the breathing as well as on the exercise.

Using small circular movements, start pushing your left sitting bone into the chair. Push it until you feel the left sitting bone as you have felt the right one.

Imagine an orange taproot growing also from this tip—one with many capillaries, which grows through the chair and sixteen inches into the ground.

> *I can't imagine this.*
> Take a piece of paper and a crayon and draw the orange-colored roots.

Now breathe into your pelvis and out through the two roots. If you succeed in feeling into these roots, you will feel your body slowly sinking down and start to calm down.

The interior of the sitting bones is, among other things, responsible for the body temperature. If you easily feel the cold, imagine making small circular movements as you slowly and patiently polish the interior of the right sitting bone with a soft white cloth. Do it from the top down, that is, from the pelvis down to the chair. Afterward, polish the left sitting bone too until it shines.

Once again scan the inside of your pelvis down to your sitting bones. Now look through your body down to your tailbone and let a taproot grow from there, just like the ones grown from your sitting bones; two to three inches in diameter and with many capillaries, it grows sixteen inches deep into the ground.

Breathe into your pelvis and out through the taproots, growing from your sitting bones and tailbone, down sixteen inches into the ground. Repeat this six times and feel the emotions during the exercise.

> *I don't feel anything.*
> It doesn't diminish the effect of the exercise. Not feeling anything only reduces your monitoring of the exercise; it might take three to six months before you can actually feel the exercise. You will, nevertheless, notice in many small details the slow change this exercise brings about.

People who regularly exercised with this tinnitus program were able to cope better with their tinnitus and with life in general. Regular exercise means doing these exercises at least five times a week.

If you want to benefit even more, tell a few people about your experience with the exercises. Talking about it helps you to make progress faster.

The more you talk about the program, the more you benefit from it. Tell your colleagues, husband, mother, brothers and sisters, and friends. The closer you are to the person you talk with about your inner feelings, the faster your progress.

Enjoy your new game.

7

....

Lesson 7

You have been working on the new exercises in Lesson 6 for two weeks or longer.

Now, choose "your" exercises from the previous six lessons. Decide how much time you want to spend exercising. You can exercise for longer than fifteen to thirty minutes a day. You will find what is appropriate for you.

You could aim to exercise twice daily for about fifteen minutes each time and to do the inner exercises whenever you find the time, for instance, while waiting around.

Exercising twice daily for fifteen minutes will slowly regenerate the whole body, and will have significant effects on your health that didn't seem possible at this stage.

If you have problems compiling your own schedule, I suggest you practice the new lesson, or the first third of it, for two weeks, and then do the rest or the second third of the lesson until you finish it. Each lesson is a self-contained and valuable training session in itself.

The Inner Healer

If you regularly exercise—the exercises must become part of your daily routine like brushing your teeth or visiting the bathroom—

you will in the long run be able to develop your own exercises, which are beneficial to you personally. That is to say, you suddenly know—by listening to your inner voice—how to change an exercise to make it a perfect fit for yourself. It is called "listening to your inner healer." This part of consciousness, this "inner healer," exists in all of us. We just aren't used to listening to this voice because there are so many external opportunities to look for help. When we suffer from a medical condition for which external sources fail to help or are insufficient (like tinnitus), we are invited to listen to our inner voice again.

Anybody who is willing to listen to this inner voice can do so. There is no special training needed. In my experience, knowing a lot can be more of a hindrance to listening to your inner voice.

To activate your inner voice, you could try saying something such as "I am willing to listen to my inner voice!" Place this sentence in a central spot where you will see it often, and repeat it three to ten times daily over a period of several weeks. You will be surprised at the results. Just repeating the sentence without giving it too much thought is best for the subconscious mind. This part of our being can't be forced to do something.

Start the exercise as usual by preparing the room. Your chair is in the preferred position; tissues, a glass of water, two tennis or massage balls, and a towel are close by; your feet are warm (with or without socks). Maybe your favorite CD is playing.

Don't forget your notebook and keep the room at a pleasant temperature.

If you have problems exercising on your own, fetch a teddy bear or a doll from one of your children or some other object that is of importance to you, and put it next to you on the sofa or chair.

How childish.
The teddy won't tell. And neither will I.

Explain the exercises to the teddy and imagine the stuffed animal doing them with you.

I'm not three anymore.

Well, yes, it's true, you aren't three anymore, but years of experience have taught me that often there still is a little three-year-old somewhere inside of us and cuddly toys, dolls, and other special objects can be helpful. I often "prescribe" teddy bears, because—as with a three-year-old—they help us to forget our loneliness. Once patients get over the embarrassment, it isn't uncommon for teddies to be invited on travels—secretly, of course.

If none of this strikes a note with you, just skip this passage. As I have said, this is a somewhat unusual book!

You will have noticed that the exercises in the book go from the lower to the upper part of the body. They start very far away from the ears and slowly work their way up to them. If doing "upper" body exercises increases your tinnitus, stay with the "lower" body exercises for the time being.

As all of these exercises increase self-healing powers, it is possible that while exercising, or on the following day, the ringing in your ears becomes louder and then softens again the day after. Participants in the courses have reported this. Don't worry! Your tinnitus won't get worse by exercising. It's possible that it might not improve, but this isn't a likely outcome.

Now stand up and knead and stretch your toes and feet as described in Lesson 2 (page 13), and then move your pelvis like a belly dancer or dance around taking care to always put your whole foot onto the floor. It shouldn't look graceful; in fact, you should clomp around clumsily.

When doing these exercises it's not important what you look like. The internal effects they have are what count. Dancing with flat feet allows the body to get rid of surplus energy and thereby make room for more invigorating energy. At home, it's important to always exercise without shoes. Initially, it's harder to perceive this exchange of energy when wearing shoes. However, once you have become more experienced you can perceive the energy with or without shoes.

Moving the Arms

If possible, remain standing. If exercising while standing is too tiring for you, please sit down. Now dance with your arms and hands.

What next?
In discos and nightclubs, I have often seen people who seem to have an innate understanding of rhythm. They dance, moving with all of their body—feet, legs, pelvis, back, arms, neck, and shoulders. Being curious by nature, I imitated these movements. Of course, I am a little shy. You are, too? We won't tell anyone, will we?

Even if you feel shy, raise your arms shoulder height and move them like the wings of a swan backward and forward.

Ouch, my neck really hurts and my arms are all heavy.

It's important to "fly" two minutes longer than seems comfortable. Then let the "lame wings" drop down, move your pelvis and toes, and let roots grow from your feet.

If you want, you can sit down now. Shake out your arms until there is a mountain of three-dimensional shapes under each arm and hand. Rest a little.

Repeat the sequence of dancing with your arms, and so on, three to five times. Then rest for five minutes.

My neck aches and my arms feel like a lead weight.
It could be that you feel your neck and arms very intensely following this exercise, which means it is an important exercise for you to do.

Increase the amount of time doing this exercise slowly.

Moving and Massaging the Hands

After a short rest sitting or lying down, sit up and look at your hands.

Open and close your hands and move the wrists until the hands become heavy. Shake out your hands and arms with imaginary sugar cubes falling from them.

Repeat the movements of the hands twice.

When I do this exercise it always reminds me that pianists live to be an usually old age. You'll most likely live to be very old as well, if you move your hands this much.

With your left hand, start massaging your right hand; massage the thumb first from the root to the tip. The thumb and index finger of your left hand move in small rotating circles slowly up to the tip of the right thumb.

Letting the Fingers Grow

Massage the thumb, three to five times, and when finished imagine your thumb growing and unfolding like a telescope until it is twice as long. Ultimately, you want to imagine your thumbs being at least sixteen inches longer.

> *Why do you always mention sixteen inches?*
> Our body is surrounded by an energy layer which some call the aura. We call it the body's energy field. You can imagine it like an egg surrounding your body and the eggshell being about sixteen inches away from you. To allow disagreeable body tension to leave our body's energy field, the extensions in our exercises should reach at least sixteen inches.

> *That all sounds very weird.*
> Go to a bookstore and look up books about the aura. The knowledge about the aura is relatively new to our culture, but other cultures have known about it for several centuries.

Now massage the right index finger as you have done with the thumb, and after four to five times, let it grow too. The index finger is the "pointing" finger; we point it at bad things, wag it at children, and use it for emphasis, so often it's particularly tense.

Then massage the middle finger and let it also unfold like a telescope. The ring finger follows. Massage and grow it like the others.

Occasionally, shake out your hands, arms, and shoulders and let them rest for a bit.

Finally, massage the little finger of your right hand. It is very important to relax the inside of the little finger. This is good for our heart. Massaging the outside of the little finger in particular loosens the tension behind our ears and on the sides of our head. Let the little finger grow two to four inches or even longer.

Whenever the ringing in your ears increases, slowly let your little toe grow, followed by your little finger, all the time breathing into your pelvis and out through the extended toes and fingers.

Finally, massage the palm of your right hand starting from the wrist to the fingers.

Always stick to the rule: The more tense you feel, the softer and shorter you should massage.

Enjoy massaging your hand. This is very beneficial to your body.

During the massage your hand may seem heavy. If this happens, shake out both hands.

When you are finished with your right hand, shake out both arms and hands; then place them in your lap and feel them. It's normal for the hands to feel different.

Rest for about two minutes. It can be difficult to sit still for two minutes without the usual distraction of food, cigarettes, or work. Do nothing for two minutes, only sit and breathe. Put your hand bowl in front of your body, breathe into your pelvis and out into your hand, which slowly sinks down along your body.

You may notice that this exercise feels almost natural now. If so, you can leave out the hand bowl; it was only an aid for the beginning.

Breathe into your pelvis as deeply as possible and let the exhalation just flow down along your body. Do this five to ten times.

After this rest period, massage your left hand and let all fingers grow.

Letting your fingers grow is one of the main exercises in helping reduce tinnitus.

Both hands are now relaxed after the massage.

Have another two-minute break breathing into the pelvis and out along the body.

Letting the Arms Grow

Shake out both arms and let them hang down alongside your body and the chair. You only move very slightly. Put your left hand onto your right shoulder joint, holding it tightly. Your right arm hangs loosely and it grows longer with every exhalation you make.

More nonsense, now what's that supposed to mean?
These unusual exercises seem to be for babies—but they help.
Hey, the shoulder starts to sink down, how come?

Breathe out an additional eight times and let the arm grow. Now stretch out both arms in front of you.

Wow, the right arm is about an inch longer, I hope it won't stay that way. Unbelievable, to be able to relax that much that you can still grow.

Now hold your left shoulder joint with your right hand and do the breathing exercise with your left arm.

I have monkey arms now; they drag along the floor.
That's how it should be.

Hold your arms straight out in front of you and check whether one is longer than the other. If so, breathe out through the shorter arm a couple of times to let it grow a bit longer.

This is a brilliant relaxation exercise that you can do with every body part—if you like it. Take the chin for example. Let it grow with every exhalation—it's a super exercise for people who grind their teeth.

Learning to Express Rage

Now that your arms and hands are nicely relaxed take a massage ball or a towel and knead it firmly. If anger starts building, feel free to say "stupid bitch" or something similar.

That's rude.
Yes, true, but you know, I won't tell anybody. We say it only secretly so nobody knows that underneath the friendly, helpful exterior lurks a King Kong, a dragon, or a monster.

Even if you only express this part of your being in secret, by using swear words or kneading something firmly, you will notice that life slowly feels better. People who answer back live longer. So, use this secret little kneading and swearing exercise to work toward having a longer and more satisfying life.

Why always these strange aggression exercises? After all,
I'm not aggressive.
Tinnitus is an auto-aggressive condition, which means that we don't aim our natural, justified aggressions at the outside world but at the inside one.

I don't feel any aggression.
Many tinnitus sufferers don't feel aggression. They might vent their aggression only in a nagging phrase like "she really could" or in an exaggerated readiness to help others. You will do yourself a big favor if you just believe me. It may even take a long time before you actually start to understand what I mean. However, in the long run, every one of these aggression exercises will enrich you.

Sing while driving in the car or at home. Shout in the car, and add a little exercise to express aggression to your daily routine.

Fortunately, you have reached the middle of the book by now; otherwise, I wouldn't dare talk about your aggression so openly. Now write the exercises from this lesson into your notebook. I hope you'll enjoy your secret-swearing exercises!

8
. . . .

Lesson 8

Y ou're at the beginning of Lesson 8.

If you have worked nonstop through the book, you'll have started fourteen weeks ago. Maybe you belong to those who have taken a little longer with each chapter and exercise. Or perhaps you have put the book aside for a while and are now picking it up again after another unsuccessful tinnitus treatment. Begin again with courage, at whatever point you are right now, and recommit to these unusual exercises on a daily basis.

Similar exercises are part of the daily routine of many Chinese adults, and are considered completely normal. We Westerners have forgotten them. In China, doctors were paid for the number of healthy people in their district. Each sick person meant a deduction from their "account." As material prosperity has and always will motivate people, the doctors quickly learned to develop methods to encourage their patients' self-healing powers.

People learned to wake up their inner doctor and healer. Even today this inner healer wants to tell us what is good for our health. If we learn to listen, it will tell us when we damage our well-being. Sometimes we're told what's bad for us through dreams, by other people, or through the newspaper and other media.

Many years ago I dreamed that the pills prescribed to me by a doctor friend were going to kill me. I immediately stopped taking them. That afternoon the doctor rang to tell me to stop taking the pills at once. He had received information that the medicine abnormally altered the blood count and should only be taken in rare circumstances and under strict medical supervision.

I had already learned to listen to my inner voice by then, and it has saved me and my family many times from making wrong decisions.

Pay attention!

Stretching Like a Cat

Arrange your room for exercising as usual.

Put on your favorite CD and start dancing like a cat. How does a cat dance? It stretches on silent paws. Stand in front of a mirror and move side to side so that your whole spine moves from right to left.

If you have a slipped disk and your doctor has prohibited sideways movements, do not do this exercise!

Raise your arms and stretch to the music; pelvis to the right, pelvis to the left; shoulders bent forward and backward. Bend the knees and repeat the movements.

That's exhausting.
Always go a few seconds longer than feels comfortable. This does not apply when you are in pain, are suffering from a serious illness, or are recuperating following an operation. Never, ever force yourself!

After dancing and stretching—it may look funny, but nobody is watching you, apart from the cat that is in the room—drop to your hands and knees and stretch like a cat.

For what reason?
The exercise strengthens your spine. It's okay if you feel a little strange or childish doing this. Be a little ridiculous. Give yourself permission.

Continue stretching, arch your back, and drop into a swayback (a convex curvature of the spine). Do this sequence three to five times, then lie down on the floor, move from side to side on your back, and pull your hair.

There's no end to her strange ideas.

Pulling the Hair

Roll from side to side and pull your hair. This may be a strange exercise, but it is important!

Some of us do this automatically or we scratch our head. It removes a lot of tension from the body, and once you get over destroying your hairdo you will really enjoy pulling at your hair.

Stay on your back for a couple of minutes. Bend your knees and put your feet flat on the floor. It might be more comfortable to push your feet into the ground, which lifts the pelvis slightly off the floor. It makes you feel more awake due to the effort it takes.

Breathe into the pelvis and out along the upper body, the pelvis, and the legs.

We will now alter the Breathing Out Using the Hand Bowl exercise (page 10) in such a way that we learn to let the breath flow down to the feet, and even sixteen inches beyond, when lying down. This exercise can be very helpful if you have trouble falling asleep.

Dealing with Resignation

It is important that we allow the exercises to help us. When we are ill and nothing seems to help, we often feel so resigned that we don't believe in anything anymore. We have to move beyond this feeling of resignation.

How can I do that?
Accept this thought, as strange or ridiculous as it might sound, and write it on a large piece of paper: "I allow myself to

let the exercises help me." Draw a picture on the piece of paper or put stickers on it—a heart, a flower, a photo of someone you love. The note is more effective when you combine the words with an image. Pin the note to a spot where you can see it several times during the day, so that the permission for something to ease your tinnitus is brought back into your memory over and over again.

Sit down on your chair and grow roots from your sitting bones and tailbone. You find this exercise on page 55—it is an important exercise.

When you have rooted the sitting bones and the tailbone, shake out your arms and hands and let cubes, balls, or pyramids fall from your fingertips. Your arms grow longer as you shake them.

Form fists with your hands and tap your lower spine, pelvic crest, buttocks, and hip joints down to the outsides of your thighs. Tap until you can really feel these parts. From time to time shake out your arms and hands.

Then form fists again and rub over the parts you have just tapped. Shake out your hands.

Now rub, tickle, and stroke those parts and feel into them: How does your body feel now? Scan your back, pelvis, stomach, and groin; feel under your pubic bone, through your hip joints to your thighs, lower legs, and feet.

Once you reach your feet, grow your toes; breathe into the pelvis and out again along the body and through the sixteen-inch long toes.

This is an important exercise.

Do the breathing seven times or if you enjoy it, do it even longer.

Rest for a couple of minutes.

Sitting on the chair, root the sitting bones and the tailbone. If you get into the habit of rooting your sitting bones and tailbone every time you sit down, your life will gain a new quality. You will become solid as a rock; you will be the center of your life, not to be overturned; you will be precise and independent.

Now imagine cleaning your pelvis tenderly and thoroughly with a white cloth until it glistens like gold or silver.

Take your imaginary cloth and wipe under the right groin, below the pubic bone, and under the left groin.

Breathe into the pelvis and imagine that the pelvis, including the groin area and the pubic bone, grow wider when you breathe in. The exhaling breath flows down along the legs.

Cleaning the Legs and the Hollows of the Knees

Continue cleaning and polishing the inside of your right thigh. In your imagination it has become a pipe and you clean the interior walls from the top down. The walls turn all light and white now.

Clean your knee with all its bones from the inside. Look at the knee as if it's an empty room. While you clean the hollow, the skin in the hollow widens as if made of rubber. It broadens until it hangs down to the floor like a sack of potatoes.

Use the cloth to clean well below the knee.

The Spot below the Knee

Right under your kneecap imagine a spot a little less than an inch wide. Then imagine the spot extending to a round window of a little more than an inch. Imagine that you are looking out through this window. Now breathe into your pelvis and out through your thigh and out through this window underneath your knee. Do this five times.

If you can still concentrate, reach into your lower leg and clean it with the cloth. Now the lower leg also turns into a pipe.

Finish by cleaning the Achilles tendon, the heel, the foot, and the toes. If you feel like it, clean between all the bones of your toes.

It might help to buy an anatomy chart or a book to look at the inside of your body. When you have cleaned all of your right leg, let the toes grow and breathe into your pelvis, which gets wider when you inhale. Your exhalation first flows through your thigh and knee, and out through the hole beneath your knee. The next time it flows further down through your lower leg and toes, and finally out through your toes, which are lengthened by sixteen inches.

Alternate between breathing out through the window below your knee and the extended toes. Then let your breath choose the path it prefers. Feel the small difference the varied exhalation makes and agree to be willing to feel such unusual new things. Everybody is able to feel it; we just haven't learned how to.

I am ready to notice unusual, subtle differences in my life, which are beneficial to me.

When you have finished with your right leg, do the same exercises with your left leg.

Closing Exercise

To finish, rub the palms of your hands together and place them over your eyes. Feel the heat and energy flow into your eyes.

Then put your fingertips together and let your hands sink down two inches in front of your body and place them on your lower belly. Enjoy how you feel.

From now on always finish exercising with this closing exercise.

Write the exercise down in your notebook.

I would like to thank you again for your courage to accompany me through this book.

9

· · · ·

Lesson 9

Y ou have probably noticed that our exercises started with the toes and legs and slowly moved up the body. For the exercises above the waist, it is important to have practiced breathing into your pelvis and out along your body (page 10). Furthermore, it is important that you have learned how to grow your toes (page 19) and to root your sitting bones and tailbone (page 55).

If those exercises aren't easy for you, choose only one of the three and practice it three times a day.

Do you work full time and don't have the time for it? Decide on three fixed times during the day: for instance, do the first exercise for two minutes before getting up, the second during your lunch break or in the restroom, and the third in the evening before dinner.

Reward yourself with three stars in your notebook each day, painted flowers, or some such-like thing for each exercise you have done.

These three exercises, together with the self-massage exercises, are the most important in the book. If you decide in favor of these three small exercises, you will have taken a significant step toward easing your tinnitus. Obviously, it would be better if you exercised more. You are the focus of each exercise.

People with tinnitus as a rule pay too little attention to themselves without noticing it. Often work, obligations, or family have become the focal points of their lives. The ringing in the ears can serve as a reminder to tinnitus sufferers to start paying more attention to themselves.

Time and again people realize that shortly before their tinnitus started, they sacrificed pleasure to fulfill their obligations, for example, by no longer playing volleyball with friends, attending a sewing circle, reading, or playing music.

If you recognize yourself in this, I suggest you take up your hobbies again.

In some cases, tinnitus diminished just by the person resuming his or her interests. Examine other aspects of your life to see if you have given up something that was important to you.

> *I am the most important person in my life.*
> Write this sentence on a piece of paper and stick it to a wall. It will bring up many reactions in you, starting from "ridiculous" and "what nonsense" to "she's right!" Allow all these reactions and try to penetrate your individual defense mechanisms to connect with your inner self. Often our duties and the supposed important needs of others lurk behind these defense guards.

In a way this book is nothing but a somewhat unusual guidebook to bringing you back into the focus of your own life. Course participants who were willing to approach their fears all benefited greatly from these small willpower exercises.

Arrange the room where you exercise as you like it best.

Stand next to the chair and move the whole body. Stretch, bend your knees, bend forward, stretch backward, do as you feel.

Then grow roots from your feet as described on page 28, and breathe into your pelvis a couple of times and out through the sixteen-inch-long roots underneath your feet.

Moving and Massaging the Shoulders

Today, you will move and massage the shoulder regions. Draw your shoulders up, backward, down, and forward. Everything hurts, how awful!

If it hurts a lot, shake out your arms, let your fingers grow. Then you raise your shoulders again and let them drop inch by inch.

Feel into the movement, even if it hurts.

Now use small movements to pull your shoulders inch-by-inch back as far as possible and then to the front until your chest is nearly hidden by your arms.

If this exercise feels uncomfortable or hurts a lot, you can be sure that this is the right exercise for you and that you need to do it.

Finish with shaking out your arms. Slowly grow your fingers and let three-dimensional shapes fall out of them. Take time to feel into your shoulders while breathing three to four times.

Put your palms high up on your chest next to your collarbone, and with your elbows draw circles in the air. First draw circles to the back, then to the front.

It is important to leave out an exercise if your doctor or physical therapist has prohibited the movement due to health reasons.

The program is effective even if you can't do all exercises.

If you are too lazy to exercise much, it is enough to do the first three exercises described in this chapter together with two others of your choice. Do these five exercises for several weeks. Then, replace the self-chosen ones with two different exercises.

Shake out your arms; the "wings" are starting to get lame. You notice this yourself and that's good. The tension in the shoulder region decreases and the arms grow tired. Go on exercising! To loosen the tension in your arms, you have to exercise a little more than you would like and enjoy.

Stretch your arms out horizontally and start drawing small circles with your hands and arms, then slowly make them bigger. When the circles are as big as they can get, change directions and let them grow smaller and smaller again.

Shake out your arms and take a rest.

Breathe into your pelvis and out through your feet and the roots attached to them.

Oops, the roots have gone.
Don't worry, that's normal. Let the roots regrow, and breathe
in and out seven to ten times.

Following the short rest, please try to recall all shoulder exercises
from your school days, your gym club, and so on.

Either practice these for five to seven minutes more or do the
small shoulder movements as described above.

When finished with the exercises, sit down on the chair and feel
your breath. As always, breathe into your pelvis and the exhalation
either takes the route along your body or through your legs and out
by the roots underneath your feet.

Start to massage, kneading the shoulders with your hands; the
left hand massages the right shoulder and vice versa. Do this under
or on top of your shirt, as you like.

How do you feel? Are the muscles hard or loose, warm or cold?

Shake out your hands occasionally.

With your left hand, massage the seventh cervical vertebra, which
sticks out at the back at the height of your shoulder girdle. Massage
the vertebra in small circular movements, knead, and rub it until
your hand and arm get tired. Shake them out.

Take a short rest and relax a bit.

Repeat the exercise using your right hand. When the right hand
gets tired too, shake it out and rest a bit.

The whole area hurts now.
Unfortunately, that's the way it is sometimes. You don't
notice the tension in the neck until you touch it. But now,
after you have massaged it, you feel every little hurtful detail
of it.

Using your left hand, massage your right shoulder, starting from
the spine to the shoulder joint and from there to the muscles of the
upper arm. Massage this part three to seven times.

When you breathe out, let your right arm and fingers grow.

Shake out the right arm occasionally and notice how it feels in relation to the left side.

Rest a little before you do the same massage with your right hand on your left shoulder, on the joint, and down to the muscles of your upper arm.

These little self-massages are very simple and beneficial for everybody. If we keep them in mind and once in a while give them as a present to ourselves or to somebody else, life becomes much less painful and more enjoyable. The body is very thankful for this type of attention.

Massaging the Outsides of the Chest

Place the palms of your hands as high up as possible underneath your armpits. Massage the right and left outsides of your chest, waist, and pelvis, five to ten times, starting from the top and moving down. At the same time breathe into the pelvis and let the little toes grow longer. Breathe out along the body and through the long toes.

Many people are very ticklish along the sides of their body. Laugh out loud, if you like, when doing the massage. The sides of our body harbor a lot of tension and anger, which in particular, is likely to be stored there.

When you have finished massaging the outsides of your upper body, enjoy the difference it makes to your physical well-being. It is amazing how much difference a small massage can make to our well-being. It helps to drink a glass of water during the massage. Allow yourself a little rest after doing the exercises and the massage, and don't start immediately with your work again. Your body is now perfectly attuned for the following visualization exercises.

The visualization exercises are essential to this book. They put the energy bodies in order and can be done anywhere. You can exercise in a waiting room, when drinking coffee, or during a work meeting—in effect, in all circumstances. All you need to do is focus your attention on the inner exercises.

Visualization Exercise Lying Down

Sit or lie down. If you lie down, put two small cushions underneath your knees for comfort. This is important for the energy to flow freely through your legs.

If needed, cover yourself with a blanket so that you don't feel chilly while exercising.

Keep your feet about sixteen inches apart. Put your hands on your lower pelvis, and breathe into it and out through extended toes. Enjoy the breath. It's a present for the body to know this breathing technique.

If you do the exercise sitting, grow roots from your sitting bones and tailbone.

The Flowing Shoulder Blades

Thus rooted, breathe calmly and imagine that your shoulder blades become pasty like dough and that they run down your back underneath your skin. Visualize this flowing down of the shoulder blades. They trickle down to your waist and further down to your buttocks. The buttocks join in this movement, and both the shoulder blades and the buttocks flow down along the backs of your thighs and the backs of your knees, down the backs of your lower legs to your heels, and out through the sixteen-inch long roots at your feet.

If your legs aren't wide enough for this gooey mass, imagine them becoming broader so everything can easily flow down the back of your body.

This exercise creates space at the back of your body. Figuratively speaking, we learn to let go of what lies behind us. If we let go of things past, we make room for what lies in front of us. With some people the exercise also warms up the body in the long run.

Finish the exercise as usual and enjoy the pleasurable feeling caused by five to fifteen minutes of this visualization exercise.

10

Lesson 10

Welcome!

You have practiced for another two weeks. Be honest with your-self: How often have you practiced? Four times, ten times, more? However many times is fine. Even if you haven't practiced at all, start working through this new lesson.

> *I am prepared to practice these new and unusual exercises*
> *for myself for fifteen minutes daily.*
> If you like, you can do them for even longer.

As stated in Lesson 9, do at least five different exercises.

The book works a lot with repetitions because it is important to realize the old patterns of your breathing, your attitude toward your body, and your thinking. It is necessary for you to find new ways of doing these things and to get used to them. And this happens through repetition and exercising!

First, always read through each new lesson. Next, practice the program you have devised for yourself for fifteen to thirty minutes. Then, start working through the new lesson.

Dancing

Sit on a comfortable chair and start with shaking your body and dancing while sitting down. Shake out your arms and upper body as if dancing to a modern rhythm. Do this for two to three minutes. Then put on a CD, stand up, and dance around.

Keep the soles of your feet flat on the ground when you dance, like tribal people do in their rituals. It relaxes your body and lengthens the tendons in your heels. If you (women) can't do this at all because you have worn high heels for many years, then for this exercise wear shoes with heels and slowly lower the height of the heel when exercising until you are able to stand barefoot again.

Always alternate between dancing and shaking out your legs and feet. Find your own rhythm. If you can't find your own rhythm, dance for three minutes and shake for one minute. Repeat this three times. If you still feel nervous, go on dancing and shaking until the restlessness has passed. Agitation is always resolved by movement, never by rest. If you feel agitated and you start with calm, inwardly directed exercises, it's like trying to stop a car going 120 miles per hour within one second. You would assault your body.

If you notice that dancing or shaking your body doesn't help at all, stop and go for a walk. My patients were very creative in inventing something to get rid of their surplus energy. One woman swept the street in front of her house. Invent something that suits you; listen to yourself.

Many thanks for your courage to time and time again try new and unusual things, such as dancing around a room all by yourself. Be thrilled with yourself; it's not a trivial thing.

As a reward, rest for several minutes doing nothing, and breathe into your pelvis and out along your body.

Whenever you exercise sitting down, always grow roots from your sitting bones and tailbone.

Take your time and calmly breathe in and out. It could be that your hands are already warm. If not, rub them together for some time. If they don't get any warmer, just continue the massage below with cool hands. Breathe into the pelvis and out along the body.

Massaging the Face, Hair, and Scalp

Put the palms of your hands on your face and rub it as if pushing around a mass of soft dough.

There's nothing to be pushed around in my face, it's all tight.

Feel how it is; it's good that way. Rub your face this way five to ten times.

Subsequently, pull your hair and move, rub, or scratch your scalp. Shake out your hands from time to time.

The ringing in the ears gets louder.

Grow your little toes and pay attention that you breathe into your pelvis. And don't worry, you already know that the ringing will diminish again after a while.

For one to two minutes, massage with the index and ring fingers the point in front of your ears, where the jaw joint is. Then massage the points an inch above and below your jaw joint, also one to two minutes each. In between, open your mouth wide and feel how the jaw moves. Open your mouth, stick out your tongue like a naughty child and quietly say, "baa."

Your hands wander from your jaw to your cheeks; knead, rub, and pinch the muscles there until your cheeks feel hot like a teenager in love. If you suffer from neuralgia in the face, don't do this exercise.

The harder the muscles feel, the softer the massage. If your cheek muscles are soft, you can pinch harder but still tenderly. Massage yourself and feel how good it is. From time to time open your mouth, stick out your tongue and say, "baa," or shout something out loud.

Now turn to your nose. Rub, push, and press your nose either with both hands or with just one hand.

The face holds a lot of tension since it is our facade, our mask, our outward appearance. When we let go of the mask, very often the tiredness of many years starts to flow away. If you feel tired, look upon it as a success and rest a little after the exercise.

It can take a long time, sometimes years, to dissolve all the old fatigue, but it's worth it. You will feel fitter and more alive. When old tension starts to dissolve, it seems like putting down a backpack after carrying it for twenty or more years. You know how it feels when you take off the backpack after a long day's hike. Exhaustion and tiredness start dropping away. Very often the face is tensed up since nursery or school days. Loosening this tension is worthwhile: you will probably look younger again.

Shake out your hands if they become heavy. Thank you. Rest a little and drink a glass of water.

Subsequently, put your hands on your chin. Defiance, imperiousness, stamina, and willpower, to name but a few, all show in the form and tension of the chin. Rub and knead it, massage it in small circular movements using your middle finger. Shake out your hands. From time to time open your mouth, stick out your tongue, and say, "baa." Let the "baa" grow bolder and insolent until you resemble a bleating sheep or a monstrous ogre.

To finish the face massage, use the palms of your hands to massage your forehead, the region around your eye sockets and cheekbones, as well as your temples and eyebrows.

To relax, let your head sink down a little and rest the eyes in the palms of your hands for one to two minutes. This feels very pleasant for the eyes. Then rest and enjoy. Watering eyes, a runny nose, or both are signs of the tension starting to dissolve.

Making the Inner Scream Audible

Now follows an exercise for the courageous and advanced learner. If you think you don't belong to this group or dare not do the exercise yet, keep it for a later date and continue with the visualization exercise for the face.

Sit on the chair and let out a small scream, and another one, and another one.

If you live in your own house and don't need to show consideration for neighbors, just shout out loud and slowly increase the volume. Open your mouth as wide as possible.

If you do have neighbors, take a sofa cushion and shout into it. Press the cushion to your mouth and shout into it; it's just as relaxing as shouting out loud. It is important to shout with your mouth wide open, because this way your jaw, chin, neck, and throat, as well as the whole lower region of your face are freed and relaxed. If all these parts are relaxed, the space of the inner and outer ears also starts to relax.

If you are well known for shouting, feelings of guilt start coming up and you may feel "I shouldn't do this." Screaming is important for your liberation. Ultimately, tinnitus is often an attempt of the body to release our silent scream. The volume of the tinnitus equals the volume of your silent scream; you can best judge that yourself. Tinnitus is a scream which is directed to the inside as that is socially acceptable. Even your partner can't hear it. You remain acceptable, and sometimes become more and more lonely because you can't bear the noise of your neighbors any longer.

The screaming exercise is important! It is also painful and costs you quite an effort to do. The whole course demands a lot of dedication from you.

Start slowly, moan a little, so you can remember and get used to the tone of your own voice.

Be gentle with yourself if you notice that you don't like hearing your voice out loud.

Take your time and release your scream. If your scream is so loud that it scares you, just feel frightened. I too am sometimes frightened by my own scream. You are on the right path if you get frightened by your own scream. Don't lose heart!

If the tinnitus increases when you scream, lower the shouting down to a whisper if need be. Sometimes we have to start very slowly and carefully.

Afterward, drink a glass of water and take a rest if you need to. Often we feel very alive and awake after shouting.

Rub your face once more and breathe into your pelvis, grow roots from your sitting bones, and breathe out through extended toes.

Inner Exercise for the Face

During this whole exercise, breathe into the pelvis and out along the body.

> *I can't do this.*
> It's normal and perfectly okay to think you can't do this. When I say that you should breathe into the pelvis at all times, it means that every time you notice that you have stopped breathing this way, you should start doing it again. You will learn to remember the right breathing technique, without having a bad conscience about having forgotten it. Just start anew, breathing in and out like this, again and again and again. Doing the daily routines with joy and awareness will increase your sense of serenity.

Sit down and imagine that your chin flows down to your pubic bone, like a rubber band or a lump of gooey dough. You can pick a different image if you like for this pasty flow between your chin and pubic bone.

You can help this visualization by putting your right hand on your pelvis when breathing in and with your left hand stroking your chin when breathing out, as if you had a pointed beard.

Exhaling, slowly stroke your "goatee" with your left hand, along your chest and down to your pubic bone. Open your mouth wide. After opening the mouth three or four times, it often happens that you start yawning because this exercise is very relaxing. Your eyes may water and your nose may start to run. Breathe out slowly and enjoy it.

This is a perfect exercise for people with tension in the neck and ears. When your chin has "flown down" like this, your exercising will slow down as a matter of course; enjoy this, too.

Shake out your hands gently and slowly; don't disturb the calmness with hectic movements.

Turn your attention to your breathing, using the familiar technique of breathing into the pelvis. Put your hands on your cheekbones as if holding your face tenderly with both hands. When you breathe out, your hands slowly glide down along your face to your lower jaw. Imagine that while you exhale a full white beard of at least sixteen inches starts to grow from your right to your left ear.

Strand by strand the beard grows and you follow its growth with your hands with every exhalation, sixteen inches down along your body. Don't take exact measurements; it could also grow twenty inches.

You continue breathing until the beard has covered your whole lower jaw from your right ear to the left ear. Sometimes the beard grows easily on the right side and not at all on the left or the other way round. It depends on which side of the body you are more aware of or which is more relaxed.

If you notice a great difference between the right and left sides of your body, you could buy a book on kinesiology. Kinesiologists specialize in the study of human movement and have developed excellent exercises to bring right and left back into balance.

Finally, shake out your hands slowly and gently; don't disturb your inner peace.

Relaxing the Tongue

This final exercise will remind you of your childhood.

Stick out your tongue. Your breath flows into your pelvis.

With every exhalation, imagine the tongue slowly uncoiling like a clown's noisemaker or a licorice wheel or a snail. With every breath out, the tongue-snail grows longer and longer until it reaches the pelvis. The shoulders sink down, the neck tension flows away, and the tension in the head starts to loosen.

This is an excellent exercise for people who have to talk a lot.

Breathe into your pelvis and out along the very, very long tongue. If your tongue gets cold, take it back into your mouth for warming up.

Finally, rub your hands together and place the palms of your hands onto the eye sockets. Let the warmth of your hands radiate into your eyes.

Let your hands sink down along your body until they rest on your thighs. Stay like this for a while, using the familiar breathing technique.

Enjoy this powerful exercise. You have come far if you have been able to follow the exercises up to this point.

Take your time to write down the exercise so that you can remember it easier.

I look forward to taking you a step further in two to three weeks.

11
. . . .
Lesson 11

By now you have exercised for at least five months, if not longer. It is perfectly fine to have taken longer than five months to reach this point. The exercises in this lesson are very varied and powerful. I have worked with them since 1982 and they remain as fresh as ever. Often I see old exercises in a completely new light. I am sometimes amazed that the depth of the exercises is never ending and if anything increases over time.

For today's session, put on a CD or listen to your favorite radio station.

Dance around for ten minutes. If you have never danced alone in a room and it seems very strange and silly, give yourself permission to be extra strange and silly and weird! You'll see that the exaggeration actually helps and that through all this weirdness you will be able to get back to your roots—to your core. The more ordered and constrained your life is, the more important is all the "strangeness" of this program. Go for it; jump over your own shadow. When you practice on your own, nobody is watching, apart from you. Be funny and liberate yourself.

After dancing for at least ten minutes, you might be a little out of breath. Sit down and observe how your whole body is agitated and alive. Feel how your breath races and your heart beats. Feel the warmth of your body. Embrace these "loud," wild emotions of your body. Many tinnitus sufferers are cautious with their bodies, however, not all are.

Allow your body to feel alive and grow roots from your sitting bones and tailbone (page 55).

When you have calmed down, start breathing into your pelvis and out along your body and feet. Breathe like this for three minutes and enjoy how peace slowly enters your body.

After a short rest, rub your hands together until they become warm. Loosen up the hands by shaking them out, and let cubes, balls, or pyramids fall out of them until your arms and hands feel relaxed.

Massaging the Eyes, Temples, and Cheekbones

Imagine that your eyes, nose, and ears are covered with a blindfold like in the game of blind-man's bluff. Massage the "covered" area by rubbing your eye sockets, eyebrows, temples, and cheekbones. Alternate between using the fingertips and the palms of your hands. If the hands feel heavy, shake them out.

After you have massaged around your eyes two to three times, cover them with the palms of your hands and let your head hang down. The fingertips rest high up on your hair. This is very relaxing for the eyes.

Enjoy your breathing. If you want to extend the relaxation to your brain and the visual nerve, imagine your eyes completely sinking into your hands.

At the beginning this feels very unfamiliar. It is a very subtle exercise, which slowly loosens a lot of tension.

Shake out your hands gently without any hectic movements. Gradually, your body is becoming more relaxed, so hectic movements would disturb your inner peace.

Take a few breaths using our special technique and if the taproots from your sitting bones and tailbone have faded away, let them regrow again.

Continue with the massage. Rub, pinch, and stroke the skin between your eyes and ears, using simple and soft movements. If your hands become heavy, shake them out.

Rest your hands in your lap and take a few breaths. Start to stretch out the inactive periods between massaging. The longer you can stay with breathing into the pelvis, the better. Through the peace, you inwardly reconnect to your core self. We lose ourselves living at a hectic pace; in calmness, we find ourselves again.

Sometimes we greatly fear peace, because it is then that we encounter our own screaming, weeping, raging self, which we have long neglected. Dare to approach yourself, even if it is painful initially to meet yourself and to see or feel all the needs that have not been satisfied for many years. Many of your fellow sufferers are masters in suppressing their own desires. Surely, you don't belong in this category? But if you do notice anything, secretly start satisfying one desire after another.

There is a way of even speeding up the process, but to some this might be a little painful. Talk to somebody about your desires, particularly about the strictly forbidden ones; it works miracles.

Massaging the Ears

Having finished the previous massage, start massaging the ears. Shake out your hands gently so that you are able to massage lightly and start with the upper rim of your ears. Pull at them, stretch and massage them until the ears become hot. Then, you rub your earlobes.

Massaging the ears has an effect on the entire body, because there are reflex points in the ears that cover the whole body. It could be that the ringing in the ears is increased through the massage, but as you already know, it will also fade again.

Put the palms of your hands over your ears and let your head drop down. Breathe into your pelvis and as usual out along your body. Enjoy the warm feeling.

Growing the Earlobes

Keep the hands over your ears and enjoy your breath. Imagine that both earlobes start to grow, first down to your shoulders, then down to your hips and along your legs until they reach to about sixteen inches below your feet. Breathe into your pelvis and out along those long earlobes.

At the beginning, this growing of different body parts was very difficult for me. If you feel the same way, you could imagine some dough or another pasty substance flowing down from your head.

Breathe into the pelvis several times and out along the earlobes. Maybe your condition temporarily worsens as your tensions in this area become noticeable for the first time. Don't let it irritate you. Continue breathing this way until the tension starts to subside again or until it is at least no worse than before.

This "increase" of the tensions is an important step in the healing process.

If you started exercising only recently, I suggest you finish with some intakes of breath into the pelvis, breathing out and down along the body.

Healing with the Inner Eyes

Do the following exercise only if your feet are warm and the exercise of growing your toes comes easily to you, because it greatly stimulates your healing powers.

Sit on the chair and let roots grow from the sitting bones and the tailbone.

Let your toes grow very long. Breathe into your pelvis and out through your legs, feet, and extended toes. Take your time and breathe at least seven times.

Close your eyes and imagine that you are capable of looking at the inside of your head. With your right and left eyes, simultaneously look toward your nose, mouth, and chin, and down into your throat.

If you notice a particularly tense spot, look at it longer with loving care. Give it special attention.

Then, wander through your whole body with your inner eyes. For people who suffer from tinnitus, it is better to pay more attention to their lower body half. Let your body call you and draw you down. "Listen" to your body and feel into the spots that are calling you and hurt you, and continue breathing into your pelvis and out through your feet.

Only when you fully understand and feel what I mean by "the energies must flow downward," are you allowed to exercise within the head and ear region. During World War II, my teacher Hetty Draayer succeeded in healing a very grave physical illness with this inner exercise, at a time when she couldn't see a doctor.

Respect your body when doing this exercise. At times it creates light in the body, as if somebody had switched on a big spotlight. Don't get frightened, light is what we are made of. Unfortunately, we sometimes have dimmed it down a little too much. If the light increases, breathe into the pelvis and send the light into all regions of the body, into the very last toe. If you feel that there still is a lot of light remaining in you, breathe it out through your extended toes.

I wish you a lot of happiness and light with this exercise.

12
· · · ·

Lesson 12

And now for a special treat . . .

You have reached the final lesson of the book.

Many times it has cost you quite an effort to get as far as this point. Thank you very much for your courage and your perseverance.

We will conclude the adventures within the inner space of your body with a very beautiful inner exercise.

The book may end here but not your exercising. It is important that you do your exercises daily, so that they will become part of your daily routine, in summer as in winter, on workdays as on Sundays.

Now, read through the lesson, do the program you have compiled for yourself once, then sit down and breathe into your pelvis and out along your legs and feet. Grow roots from the sitting bones and the tailbone. Whenever you sit down, grow roots from these three points. You will be directly connected with your core and will become as solid as a rock.

Clean under your groin and pubic bone as described in Lesson 4 (page 38). Imagine your legs turning into pipes and grow your toes. The breath flows into the pelvis and out through the legs, feet, and extended toes into the universe.

Light Healing the Ear

Wipe out your pelvis very lovingly with the imaginary soft white cloth, and clean once under your groin.

Imagine that a huge ear sprouts from the right side of your pelvis. The corresponding part of the inner ear is nestled inside your pelvis.

Now, the left inner ear grows within the left side of your pelvis and the earflap grows on the left exterior. It is as if your ears, including the inner ears, have slipped down to the height of your pelvis.

Attach a small but bright spot lamp at the back of your pelvis, right above your tailbone. Let the light beam flow through the whole inner ear: from the eardrum it passes the hammer, anvil, and stirrup and then flows through the auditory canal, the light illuminating everything from there to the cochlea. You breathe into your pelvis and out through your feet.

This exercise relaxes your whole ear.

After illuminating every last corner of the inner ears in your pelvis, send the light to the outer ears on the outsides of your pelvis and subsequently also behind the inner ears. A person with tinnitus "has a lot of slyness behind her or his ears" as the German saying goes (meaning the person is a sly old dog). Unfortunately, the individual doesn't know it her- or himself and therefore can't feel the repercussion of all this tension behind the ears.

Sun and Moon Exercise

Now imagine that the right ear at your pelvis is a window.

The sun is sixteen inches away from the window. Its beam shines onto the whole outer ear and then flows through the auditory canal into the inner ear in your pelvis.

The light fills all corners of your left and right inner ears and pelvis, and then flows out through the left ear on your pelvis. The beam also embraces the left outer ear and then flows a good sixteen inches further.

This exercise creates warmth, alertness, and light in you.

If your ears are inflamed and in need of cold and peace, you should do the visualization from left to right and use moonlight rather than sunshine. In this case, the moonbeam is sixteen inches away from the left side of your pelvis and shines onto the outer ear and into the inner ear of the pelvis. Then it flows out through the right outer ear and a further sixteen inches from there.

The exercise with the moon is a wonderful ancient one, which can also be used to fall asleep (again) when you lie awake at night.

Don't be tempted to start with this exercise because it apparently fits your tinnitus problem perfectly. You will not benefit from it as much initially as you will now.

All previous lessons serve as preparation for this powerful and light-flooded healing exercise. It takes time, effort, and practice to work your way through the Tinnitus Alleviation Therapy program, but once you do the harvest will be yours.

Please accept my sincere thanks.

Afterword

With this book I want to encourage you to find your own path for healing or easing your tinnitus. People are unique and so is their tinnitus.

Participants in my Tinnitus Alleviation Therapy (TAT) courses had most creative and unusual ways to help reduce their levels of stress and relieve their tinnitus, among them: sweeping the street, cleaning windows, sticking unwashed wool into the ears, sleeping with unwashed wool in the ears, wearing only woolen clothes, or taking a walk under high-voltage power lines! Many people found kneading dough was a way that proved to be successful.

Invent your own solutions and be audacious.

In order to take full advantage of this book, you need to exercise daily, even if you have completed all the exercises once.

Should you be among the fortunate people who completely get rid of the ringing noise, continue exercising.

For many TAT participants and people receiving individual TAT instruction, the ringing in the ears lost its significance and they used it as a sign of their well-being. If it increased, they knew it was again time to take more care of themselves.

You can exercise on your own or together with others, but not with other tinnitus sufferers.

Why is that so? With tinnitus sufferers, the energy flow within the body has been misaligned upward. Exercising with others who suffer from the same medical condition intensifies this phenomenon unfavorably. It is known that people who work with tinnitus sufferers are at risk of also developing a ringing in the ears.

When doing this self-healing program in groups, it is advisable to be supervised by qualified people. It is good to have a course leader, or therapist, who guides participants through the exercises and stabilizes the group's energies. The leader should be trained in the exercises and should have practiced them themselves for at least one and a half years.

It is important that course leaders be well advanced in their own daily exercising before they offer such courses. It's not enough to read the exercises out loud. A course leader needs to be able to feel the exercises in his or her own inner space, otherwise he or she isn't capable of leading the group in the restructuring of the energy bodies.

The group sessions should be held at intervals of two to three weeks or over three weekends, each of them two weeks apart. It is necessary to have the appropriate time in between sessions for participants to work on the exercises in their self-compiled programs.

These exercises are specifically designed for tinnitus sufferers, but many of us are familiar with some of the mental conditions described in the book without suffering from ringing in the ears.

Everybody encountering this book is invited to take an adventure through it and make use of these initially strange-seeming, very ancient exercises.

I hope that my book will contribute to relieving the condition of many tinnitus sufferers.

Take good care of yourself! That's the most important step toward your healing.

If the exercise program is of help to you, please pass it on.

Recommended Reading

Chang, Stephen. *Complete System of Self-Healing Internal Exercises.* San Francisco: Tao Publishing, 1994.

Diamond, John. *Your Body Doesn't Lie.* New York: Grand Central Publishing, 1989.

Draayer, Hetty. *Das kosmische Auge: Wie wir den Weg der inneren Heilung gehen* [in German and Dutch]. Munich: Kösel Verlag, 2002.

——. *Finde dich selbst durch Meditation* [in German and Dutch]. Darmstadt: Schirner Verlag, 2007.

Lowen, Alexander. *Bioenergetics: The Revolutionary Therapy that Uses the Language of the Body to Heal the Problems of the Mind.* New York: Arkana Publishing, 1994.

Lowen, Alexander, Leslie Lowen, and Walter Skalecki. *The Way to Vibrant Health.* Alachua, FL: Bioenergetic Press, 2003.

Ohashi, Wataru, and Kan Okano. *Beyond Shiatsu: Ohashi's Bodywork Method.* New York: Kodansha America, Inc., 2003.

Resource Organizations

American Tinnitus Association
522 S.W. Fifth Avenue, Suite 825
Portland, OR 97204
Phone: (800) 634-8978
Website: www.ata.org

British Tinnitus Association
Ground Floor, Unit 5
Acorn Business Park, Woodseats Close
Sheffield, S8 0TB England
Phone: 0044 (0)114 250 9922
Website: www.tinnitus.org.uk

Institut Maria Holl GmbH
An den Frauenbrüdern 2
52064 Aachen, Germany
Phone: 0049 (0)241 46372213
Website: www.tinnitus-coach.eu
Email: service@tinnitus-coach.eu

International Institute for Bioenergetic Analysis
Website: www.bioenergetic-therapy.org

**Multidisciplinary Tinnitus Clinic
at the University of Regensburg**
Phone: 0049 (0)941 944-9410
Email: info@tinnituszentrum-regensburg.de
Website: www.tinnituszentrum-regensburg.de

Index

Dedications, 5
Defense mechanisms, 74
Dependence, 33, 55
Desires, 89
Displays. *See* Symbols.
Distractions, 3
Dizziness, 27–28
Draayer, Hetty, 91
Drawings, 18, 24, 28, 43, 56, 70

E

Ears and earlobes, 84, 89, 94–94
   "lengthening" of, 90
Emotions. *See* Feelings.
Energy field, 20, 27–28, 56, 63
Energy, life, 2, 3, 10, 14, 20, 24,
   28–29, 35, 46, 78, 91, 97–98
Energy pathways. *See* Meridians.
Exercises, 2–6, 18, 19, 21, 24,
   31–32, 35–36, 41, 49, 57, 59,
   67, 69–70, 73, 75, 79, 87, 93,
   97
  anger, 33, 66
  bioenergetic, 2, 97–98
  breathing, 3, 8–9, 16, 18, 38,
   39, 20, 22, 24, 27, 29, 37–38,
   42–43, 44, 54, 55, 64, 69, 71,
   73, 76, 78, 84–85
  closing, 72
  drawings of, 18, 24, 43, 56,
   70
  inner, 3, 90–91, 94
  loosening up, 25–26, 33–35,
   42–44
  relaxation, 65, 84, 85–86
  repetitions of, 79
  rubbing/scratching, 35, 81
  talking about, 57

visualization, 19, 77–78, 84,
   85–86, 90–91, 94–95
writing down, 12, 18, 24, 37,
   45, 54, 72, 86
Exhalation, 20, 24, 27, 55, 65, 71,
   72
Exhaustion, 9, 11, 15, 37
Eyes, 82, 86, 88–89

F

Fears, 3, 35, 38, 46, 74
Feelings, 4, 16, 17, 19, 23–25,
   32–34, 37, 49–50, 56, 57, 66
  angry, 32–34, 45, 66
  expressing, 32–34, 45, 66,
   82–83
  guilty, 32, 33, 83
  negative, 50
  restoration of, 16, 23–24
  suppressed, 2, 82–83, 89
Feet, 3, 8, 11, 13–16, 19–20, 23,
   24, 25, 27, 80
  soles, 28, 43
Fingers, 63–65
  "lengthening" of, 63–65

G

Groin, 36, 45–46, 93
Growing Roots from the Sitting
   Bones and the Tailbone
   (exercise), 55–56, 73, 78, 80,
   88, 90, 93
Growing Taproots Out of the
   Soles of Your Feet (exercise),
   28, 43, 46, 74

H

Hair, pulling of, 69, 81

About the Author

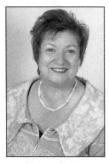 Psychotherapist and alternative medicine prac-
titioner **Maria Holl** from Aachen, Germany,
gathered knowledge from many different areas
before she developed her outstanding program
eighteen years ago. Using this unique synthesis of
Chinese medicine, massage, and psychotherapy,
her patients succeed in reducing their ringing in
the ears—or even get rid of it altogether.

During the 1970s Maria Holl began to combine knowledge from
very different fields. After studying social pedagogy and social work,
she was certified in bioenergetic analysis—a body-orientated form of
psychoanalysis—at the Institute of Bioenergetic Analysis, founded
by Alexander Lowen, M.D., in New York. For a further fifteen years,
she studied a combination of Western and Eastern techniques like
meditation and traditional Chinese medicine with the Dutch meditation teacher and author Hetty Draayer, who lived in Indonesia for
many years. Her teacher in shiatsu was Wataru Ohashi.

Tinnitus Alleviation Therapy combines physical exercises to
mobilize the body, massage to activate the blood circulation and
the immune system, and exercises which originate in the Chinese
knowledge of the meridians, or *chi*. Even though the exercises originate in very different areas, their combination is far from arbitrary.

They are the result of a long learning process, which, in 1995, enabled Maria Holl to develop her unique therapy. It has helped many tinnitus sufferers since.

Since 1981 Maria Holl has her own practice where she works as psychotherapist, consultant, and meditation teacher. She has conducted individual and group courses in Tinnitus Alleviation Therapy for children and adults since 1995.

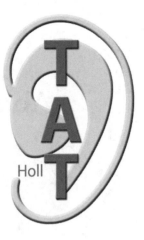